Acclaim for *COPD: Answers to Your Questions*

"In this clearly written and easy-to-understand book, Dr. Mahler provides the answers to questions doctors often hear from COPD patients and their families. The answers are very practical and will be helpful for many patients suffering from the disease."

Nicholas S. Hill, MD
Chief, Division of Pulmonary, Critical Care and Sleep Medicine
Tufts Medical Center
Professor of Medicine, Tufts University School of Medicine
Boston, Massachusetts

"This book is an excellent and unique guide for patients and their families to better understand COPD. It provides essential information with original vignettes and practical instructions. Both patients and physicians will get helpful suggestions from its well-organized content."

Toru Oga, MD
Department of Respiratory Care and Sleep Control Medicine
Graduate School of Medicine
Kyoto University, Kyoto, Japan

"All too often, medical care for COPD focuses on risk avoidance and medications, leaving too little time for answering the important questions that patients or their family members might have. This short book, written by an internationally recognized authority on COPD, answers many of these questions. The insights provided, which reflect years of experience by an excellent clinician, should prove very useful for those affected directly or indirectly by this common disease."

Richard L. ZuWallack, MD
Clinical Professor of Medicine
University of Connecticut Health Center, Pulmonary Medicine
St. Francis Hospital and Medical Center
Hartford, Connecticut

D1496425

"Dr. Mahler provides a powerful but simple tool for patients and their families to understand symptoms, why they happen, and available treatments. Understanding and awareness are key steps for creating a meaningful lifestyle in the context of having COPD."

Roberto Benzo, MD, MS
Associate Professor of Medicine,
Mindful Breathing Laboratory,
Mayo Clinic,
Rochester, Minnesota

COPD

Answers to Your Questions

COPD

Answers to Your Questions

DONALD A. MAHLER, MD

Two Harbors Press
Minneapolis, MN

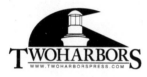

Two Harbors Press
322 First Avenue N, 5th floor
Minneapolis, MN 55401
612.455.2293
www.TwoHarborsPress.com

ISBN-13: 978-1-63413-297-8
LCCN: 2014922778

Distributed by Itasca Books

Typeset by James Arneson

Printed in the United States of America

To Richard A. Matthay, MD, and Jacob Loke, MD,
mentors during my fellowship training at Yale.
I am forever grateful for your guidance.

Contents

Acknowledgments

These chapters have been revised many times after discussions with two individuals who have COPD as well as colleagues who work at Dartmouth-Hitchcock Medical Center.

I am grateful for the insights provided by Victoria Cameron, who has alpha-1 antitrypsin deficiency emphysema and has worked as a patient advocate, and Peter Hottenstein, who had severe COPD and worked as a pharmacist. Mr. Hottenstein reviewed several chapters before he passed away.

Special thanks to Nicola J. Felicetti, RN, BS, continuing care manager in cystic fibrosis; Xan P. Gallup, RRT, RN, AE-C, pulmonary nurse educator; Heidi A. Pelchat, RRT, RCP, pulmonary rehabilitation coordinator; Sharona Sachs, MD., interim chief of the Section of Palliative Care; and Laurie A. Waterman, RRT, MS, CCRP, pulmonary research coordinator. These dedicated professionals provided helpful comments and suggestions from their unique perspectives.

I appreciate the creative efforts of Kyle Morrison (kyle@leftrightcreative.com) who designed simple and instructive graphics that illustrate important points in the text.

From my perspective, the collective input from these individuals ensures that readers receive practical information that will positively affect their daily lives.

Preface

E very day that I see someone who has chronic obstructive pulmonary disease (COPD) in my medical practice, I am reminded that the majority of these individuals and their concerned family members have many questions. These generally focus on three important uncertainties:

- What is COPD?
- Are treatments available to help me or my loved one breathe easier?
- Will my breathing, or the breathing of my loved one, get worse?

In response to these and many other questions, I have written this book to provide answers for those 24 million Americans who have COPD as well as for their family members. Each of the nine chapters focuses on a major challenge faced by someone with COPD. The reader can choose to read the book from start to finish, or may select the chapter with their topic of interest. For example, the individual may wish to learn about oxygen therapy specifically because it has been prescribed recently. However, the reader may then seek out information about inhaler medications, pulmonary rehabilitation, as well as other treatments to relieve breathing difficulty.

My daily interactions with individuals who have COPD reveal that spouses, partners, and adult children are quite interested to learn about this disease so that they can "help their loved one." Many family members report that they wish there was something they could do to help out. This book provides practical information for all interested parties.

A unique feature of the book is that each chapter begins with a vignette describing one of my patients with COPD.

The vignette provides a brief description of the situation experienced by that individual. Next, information is provided that addresses that particular situation. Key points of the chapter are then summarized. Finally, a follow-up to the vignette reports what actually happened to the individual described at the beginning of each chapter.

CHAPTER 1

What Is COPD?

Vignette

Mary is a sixty-three-year-old woman who made an appointment with her doctor because she wanted to know why she was having shortness of breath for the past six months. She found that it was "hard to breathe" when doing housework, gardening, and walking her dog. Mary had smoked one pack of cigarettes for thirty-nine years, but had quit smoking ten years ago. A few years back, she retired as an occupational therapist. She had no history of any lung disease, and was being treated for a "low thyroid" and high cholesterol. An older brother was diagnosed with emphysema a few years ago. Mary told her neighbor that she felt like the woman in the television advertisement who described how her breathing was "like an elephant sitting on my chest."

Introduction

COPD is an abbreviation for chronic obstructive pulmonary disease.

Definition of COPD

"A preventable and treatable disease characterized by airflow obstruction that is usually progressive and associated with an enhanced chronic inflammatory response in the airways and the lung to noxious particles and gases."[1]

What does this definition mean? Like many other chronic conditions, inflammation (redness and swelling) plays a key role in the development of this disease. It is well known that cigarette smoking is the major cause of COPD. However, only about one out of five individuals who smoke a pack or more of cigarettes per day for twenty or more years actually develops COPD.

Two important factors determine whether someone "gets" COPD:

- long-term inhalation of cigarette smoke, dust, fumes, and/or fibers
- a genetic (hereditary) susceptibility to the harmful effects of these airborne irritants

To understand how COPD develops, it is important to consider both the environment and the response of the individual person.

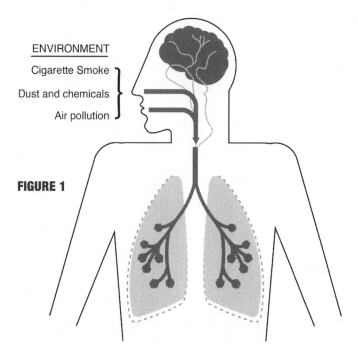

ENVIRONMENT
Cigarette Smoke
Dust and chemicals
Air pollution

FIGURE 1

Environment

From the perspective of our lungs, the environment is the air that we breathe. Although cigarette smoke is the major risk factor for COPD, the total amount of "bad air" over time, or inhaled airborne irritants, is most important. Two examples of such irritants are:

- dust and other particulate matter inhaled by a construction worker
- smoke from burning wood and fuels inhaled by a woman in a developing country while preparing meals indoors

The Individual

Each of us is born with unique physical characteristics, such as the color of our hair and eyes, which we inherit from our parents. If you smoke cigarettes or inhale airborne irritants, your individual genes influence whether you will develop COPD. It would be great if doctors could take a sample of saliva or blood and identify those individuals who are at risk for developing breathing problems. At the present time, only one genetic factor—called alpha-1 antitrypsin deficiency (abbreviated A1AT)—has been identified for COPD.

The alpha-1 antitrypsin protein is made in the liver, released into the blood, and circulates in blood vessels of the lungs. Its main purpose is to protect lung tissue from destruction by enzymes released from inflammatory cells. If the A1AT protein is blocked in the liver and does not reach the lungs, enzymes will destroy the lung tissue, resulting in emphysema. This typically occurs in the lower parts of the lungs in those with A1AT deficiency. Fortunately, a blood test can be performed to diagnose this deficiency. This test will be discussed later in this chapter.

What Are the Different Types of COPD?

To understand the two types of COPD—chronic bronchitis and emphysema—it is important to consider the anatomy of the respiratory system. Called the "tracheobronchial tree" because the structures appear like an upside-down tree, the trachea, or windpipe, is the trunk of the tree; the airways include primary and secondary bronchi that are the branches of the tree; the airways divide numerous times and end in alveoli, or air sacs, which serve as the leaves of the tree. The air we breathe contains 21 percent oxygen, which passes through the airways to reach the air sacs. Oxygen then crosses a thin membrane to enter the blood, whereas carbon dioxide, a waste product of our body, transfers from the blood into the air sacs and is eliminated in the air that we exhale.

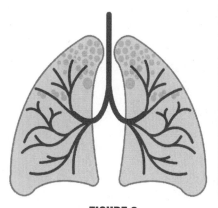

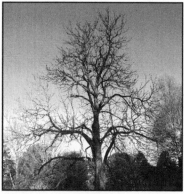

FIGURE 2   **FIGURE 3**

Due to genetic factors that are not completely understood, the toxic effects of cigarette smoke and airborne irritants may predominantly affect breathing tubes (airways), causing chronic bronchitis, *or* may predominantly affect air sacs (alveoli) and adjacent blood vessels, causing emphysema. Many individuals with COPD have features of both chronic bronchitis and emphysema.

What Is Chronic Bronchitis?

The major changes of chronic bronchitis are illustrated in Figure 4. Chronic bronchitis includes:

- inflammation of the inner lining that causes the airway wall to thicken
- mucus, a thick substance typically white or gray in color, produced by glands inside the airways; the mucus may turn yellow or green with an infection

Both the thickened airway wall and mucus inside the airway block, or obstruct, the flow of air when breathing out.

Normal Breathing Tube   Narrowed Breathing
                               Tube with COPD

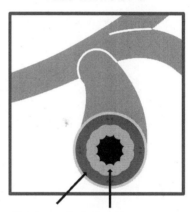

FIGURE 4   Wall Is Thickened   Mucus

Definition of Chronic Bronchitis

Cough productive of mucus on most days for at least three months per year for two years in a row.

Your doctor can make this diagnosis by simply asking you how often you cough up mucus. However, not all individuals who have chronic bronchitis develop COPD. This may seem confusing, but a person can have chronic bronchitis without having airflow obstruction on breathing tests. This is one reason why it is important that breathing tests be performed to accurately diagnose whether someone has COPD.

What Is Emphysema?

In simple terms, emphysema means that parts of the lung have been destroyed.

The top right of Figure 5 shows the destruction of multiple air sacs (alveoli) compared to the normal appearance of air sacs at the bottom right, which resemble a cluster of grapes.

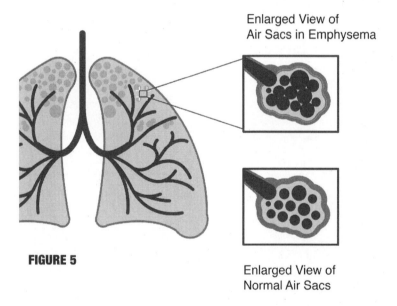

Enlarged View of
Air Sacs in Emphysema

FIGURE 5

Enlarged View of
Normal Air Sacs

These destructive changes lead to three major problems:

- The lungs lose the ability to allow oxygen to transfer from air sacs into the blood.

- Some attachments that keep the airways open are destroyed, resulting in the collapse of breathing tubes during exhalation.
- The air that is normally exhaled remains trapped in the lungs.

This trapped air causes the lungs to enlarge, or hyperinflate, as shown in Figure 6. This hyperinflation causes the muscle fibers of the diaphragm to shorten and adds an elastic load as though an elastic band has been wrapped around the chest. Hyperinflation is an important concept to understand because it is a major factor that causes breathing discomfort. Hyperinflation is also why you may feel like you cannot get enough air in.

Hyperinflation

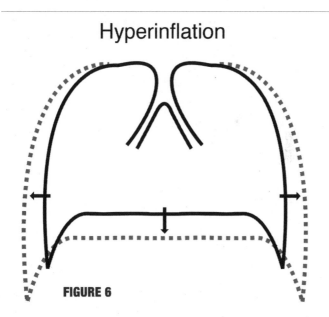

FIGURE 6

The solid outline shows the normal position of the chest wall and diaphragm muscle, whereas the dashed outline shows hyperinflation of the lungs, which causes shortened muscle fibers and elastic loading.

What Is Airflow Obstruction?

COPD is characterized by airflow obstruction—a medical term that means reduced flow of air during exhalation. The factors that cause airflow obstruction are mucus inside the airway, thickening of the airway wall, and constriction, or tightening, of the muscle that wraps around our breathing tubes. In healthy individuals, this bronchial smooth muscle is relaxed, and so the individual has no problem exhaling air. However, in those who have COPD or asthma, the muscle may be constricted at rest and tighten even more with physical activity, when inhaling cold air, dust, cleaning sprays, and fumes, or with a chest infection. This narrowing of the airways causes air to flow out of your breathing tubes at a slower pace than normal.

Why is this information so important? Because different treatments target the different mechanisms that cause airflow obstruction. These treatments will be presented in Chapter 4: Can You Help Me Breathe Easier?

How Is Airflow Obstruction Diagnosed?

Breathing tests, also called pulmonary function tests (PFTs), are required to diagnose airflow obstruction. Figure 7 (next page) shows a test that measures the amount of air exhaled after taking in a full deep breath.

How Is COPD Diagnosed?

Airflow obstruction is necessary to diagnose someone with COPD. Once this has been shown, your doctor will consider your symptoms, smoking history, any occupational exposures, family history of any respiratory illness, and the results of your physical examination, breathing tests, and chest x-rays to decide whether you have COPD. Some individuals may have features of both asthma and COPD.

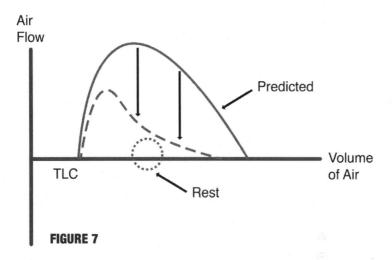

FIGURE 7

After a person takes a full deep breath to total lung capacity (TLC), he/she exhales hard and fast until all of the air is out. The curve labeled "Predicted" is considered normal in a healthy person. The dashed curve shows that exhaled airflow is reduced below the predicted curve as indicated by the arrows pointing downward.

In general, the diagnosis of COPD is based on three factors:

- shortness of breath with activities and/or chronic cough
- previous or current cigarette smoking and/or inhalation of airborne irritants like dust or fumes
- airflow obstruction on breathing tests

How Is Alpha-1 Antitrypsin Deficiency Diagnosed?

A blood test can measure the level of the A1AT protein to look for a deficiency. In general, A1AT deficiency should be suspected in a person who develops the emphysema type of COPD at an early age (usually under forty-five years of age) with minimal or no risk factors for developing emphysema, with emphysema in the lower parts of the lung as indicated by a chest x-ray or CT scan, and with unexplained liver disease.

In the United States, this genetic defect is most frequent if your ancestors were from Europe. It is recommended that the A1AT level be measured in "symptomatic adults with emphysema, COPD, or asthma with airflow obstruction that is not completely reversible after aggressive treatment with bronchodilators."[2]

If you fit one or more of the above situations, you should ask your doctor about ordering a blood test to measure your A1AT level.

Why is it important to know this? First, the A1AT protein can be given through a plastic tube placed in an arm vein once a week to prevent emphysema from worsening. This is called augmentation therapy. Second, because A1AT deficiency is hereditary, you should inform any children and grandchildren if you have this deficiency so that they can be tested to find out if they are at risk for this form of emphysema or if they are a carrier of the gene.

Key Points

1. If you experience shortness of breath with your activities, do not assume that you are just getting old or are out of shape. Tell your doctor!
2. COPD is diagnosed by a combination of symptoms (mainly breathlessness and cough), a history of smoking and/or inhaling airborne irritants, and airflow obstruction on breathing tests.
3. Once COPD is diagnosed, there are many treatments that can help your breathing.

Follow-Up Vignette

After examining Mary, the doctor ordered breathing tests. These tests were done at the local hospital. The next day, Mary's doctor called and told her that the test results were lower than expected, and that COPD was the cause of her shortness of breath. The doctor suggested that she come in for an appointment the following week to discuss different treatments for her COPD. Mary was relieved to know that there was a reason for her breathing difficulty, and planned to call her brother to ask what medications he was taking for his COPD.

Patient and Family Information

The mission of the **COPD Foundation** is to develop and support programs that improve the quality of life through research, education, early diagnosis, and enhanced therapy for persons whose lives are impacted by chronic obstructive pulmonary disease.

Website: www.copdfoundation.org
Phone: 866-316-2673

The **Alpha-1 Association** is a member-based non-profit organization dedicated to identifying those affected by alpha-1 antitrypsin deficiency and improving the quality of their lives through support, education, advocacy, and participation in research.

Website: www.alpha1.org
Phone: 800-521-3025

CHAPTER 2

Why Am I Short of Breath?

Vignette

F ive years later, Mary is now sixty-eight years old and notes that her "breathing is getting harder." Carrying grocery bags up two steps into her house and playing with her four- and six-year-old grandchildren have caused breathing difficulty and the need to stop to "catch her breath." These same activities did not cause any problem just one year ago. Mary uses a long-acting inhaled bronchodilator in the morning along with albuterol as needed before doing activities that make her short of breath. However, she is concerned that her COPD has become worse.

Introduction

We normally breathe ten to twelve times every minute without even thinking about it. Thus, the act of breathing is an unconscious one. A group of nerves called the respiratory center is located at the base of the brain, called the brainstem, and provides an automatic command to breathe. The respiratory center is a "pacemaker for breathing" as it sends signals (represented by the downward arrow in Figure 8) through nerves to the breathing muscles that control how often and how deeply we breathe. This process is similar to a group of nerves in the heart that controls how often the heart beats.

However, you can also voluntarily control your breathing. In other words, the brain can override the automatic control. For example, you can hold your breath for as long as possible,

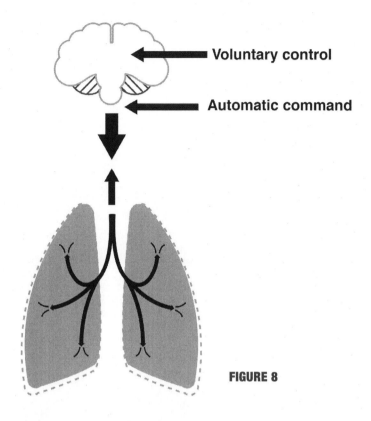

Voluntary control

Automatic command

FIGURE 8

as many of us likely tried as kids, or breathe out forcibly to blow up a balloon. No other part of our body is under both automatic and voluntary control.

What Is Dyspnea?

Dyspnea is a medical term that describes breathing discomfort or difficulty. To simplify communication, many doctors use words or phrases like "breathlessness" or "shortness of breath" rather than dyspnea. In essence, dyspnea is a complaint by an individual that his or her breathing does not feel "right" or normal.

Definition of Dyspnea

"A subjective experience of breathing discomfort that consists of qualitatively distinct sensations that vary in intensity."[3]

To understand how dyspnea develops, it is important to consider how our respiratory system and brain communicate (see Figure 9). Our body has numerous receptors, or sensors, that send signals via nerves to the brain. As an example, if you stub your toe, pain receptors send electrical signals through nerves to the brain to inform you that the toe hurts. Similarly, various receptors located in the neck, lungs, and chest muscles can be activated to cause breathing discomfort.

One of these receptors is called the carotid body, a group of nerves located where the carotid artery divides in the neck. The right and left carotid bodies detect the level of oxygen in the blood that is going to the brain. If the blood oxygen level is low for whatever reason, the carotid bodies send electrical signals through nerves to the brain.

The brain responds by sending signals to our breathing muscles in an attempt to compensate, or increase, the oxygen level and increase breathing.

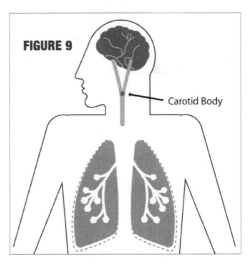

FIGURE 9

Carotid Body

In addition to the carotid bodies, there are receptors in our airways, lungs, and chest muscles. When a condition stimulates one or more of these receptors, electrical signals are sent to the brain to indicate breathing difficulty. Figure 10 provides examples of different conditions that may activate receptors in our body to cause breathing difficulty.

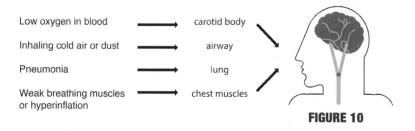

Low oxygen in blood ⟶ carotid body

Inhaling cold air or dust ⟶ airway

Pneumonia ⟶ lung

Weak breathing muscles or hyperinflation ⟶ chest muscles

FIGURE 10

Why is this important to know? Quite simply, our nervous system enables communication between parts of our body and the brain. It is important to remember that different conditions can activate different receptors to cause breathing difficulty, and feeling short of breath may not always be due to a low blood oxygen level.

If you have COPD, or are a family member of someone with COPD, you might assume or believe that a low oxygen level is the main reason for breathing difficulty. Certainly, a low oxygen level can cause the feeling that it is hard to breathe. However, if you have pneumonia and are given oxygen to breathe, your breathing may not return to normal. Why not? For the reason described above: different receptors in the airways, lungs, and chest muscles may cause you to have breathing difficulty.

What Are the Different Experiences of Dyspnea?

Over the years, researchers have learned that there are different experiences of breathing discomfort just like there are different types of pain.[4] For a long time, the medical profession considered only the intensity of breathing discomfort. However, you may also experience breathing difficulty to be unpleasant. Depending on the situation, the feeling of not being able to get enough air in can cause you to feel anxious or even have a panic response. It is important that someone with COPD, as well as family members, recognize that individuals may experience breathing difficulty in different ways.

Experiences of Dyspnea

Intensity: How intense or strong is your breathing?

Unpleasantness: How unpleasant or uncomfortable is your breathing?

Impact or burden on daily activities: How does dyspnea affect your quality of life and your ability to perform daily activities?

How Does Dyspnea Impact Daily Activities?

Breathing difficulty usually impacts a person's quality of life and their ability to perform daily activities. Figure 11 describes the frequency of breathlessness reported by over 3,000 persons with COPD living in the United States, Canada, and six European countries when doing five different activities.[5]

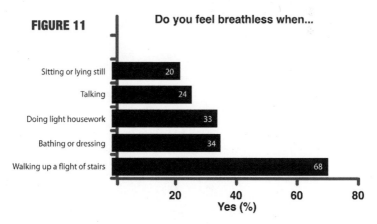

FIGURE 11

Do you feel breathless when...

Activity	Yes (%)
Sitting or lying still	20
Talking	24
Doing light housework	33
Bathing or dressing	34
Walking up a flight of stairs	68

The numbers at the right of the bars represent the average percent of individuals who answered "yes" to feeling breathless upon doing the specific activity.

The challenge of doing one or more of these daily activities may lead to frustration. To minimize or avoid breathing discomfort, the person with COPD commonly reduces or even stops doing certain tasks. If an inactive lifestyle continues, the individual becomes deconditioned or out of shape and may gain weight. Both deconditioning and weight gain add to, or complicate, any breathing difficulty. If this process continues, the patient may become depressed and choose to stay at home rather than be active. Social isolation further impacts the person's quality of life.

Key Points

1. Dyspnea is a medical term for breathing discomfort or difficulty.
2. A feeling of shortness of breath is not always due to a low oxygen level.
3. Breathing difficulty can impact a person's ability to perform daily activities and affect quality of life. Over time, this may cause frustration and lead to feelings of anxiety and/or depression.

Follow-Up Vignette

Although Mary was concerned that her COPD was getting worse, her breathing tests, chest x-ray, and oxygen levels were unchanged compared with one year ago. After her doctor asked more questions, Mary revealed that she had tripped and fallen about nine months ago. An x-ray at the time showed that her arm was fractured, and she had to wear a sling for six weeks. Mary was forced to reduce her physical activities. Over time, she lost some of her fitness and gained seven pounds. Both of these factors contributed to an increase in breathing difficulty.

Her doctor recommended that she participate in a pulmonary rehabilitation program and lose weight. Mary told her doctor that she would start an exercise program and a diet on her own.

At a follow-up appointment a few months later, Mary reported gradual but steady improvement in her breathing and stamina, and she had lost four pounds. She expressed confidence that her breathing would continue to improve, but realized it would take more time to get back to her pre-fracture fitness level.

CHAPTER 3

Can You Help Me Quit Smoking?

Vignette

James is a seventy-two-year-old man who was diagnosed with COPD four years ago. His family doctor prescribed an inhaler containing albuterol and ipratropium (brand name: Combivent) to use three to four times a day. Although this medication helped his breathing, James continued to smoke one pack of cigarettes each day. Although most of his friends had quit smoking, James's younger brother continued to smoke. Both James and his brother enjoyed smoking together, especially when they went camping and fishing.

About three months ago, James cut down to ten cigarettes each day after being nagged by his children during the holidays. However, he became very irritable and argued with everyone. James felt better when he went back to smoking a pack per day, but also felt guilty because he knew that he was disappointing his family.

At the next visit with his primary care doctor, James asked what treatments could help him quit smoking.

Introduction

It is essential that anyone who has COPD not smoke cigarettes and avoid inhaling irritants such as dust, smoke, and fumes in the air. By quitting smoking, you slow down the decline in your lung function, lower your chances of getting heart disease or lung cancer, and reduce your chances of getting osteoporosis, or thinning of the bones. In addition, your clothes will no longer smell like cigarette smoke.

The greatest barrier for anyone to quit smoking is addiction to the nicotine in cigarette smoke. Nicotine addiction appears to be greatest if you have smoked for many years, if you smoke daily, and if you smoke within thirty minutes of getting up in the morning. The degree of nicotine dependence predicts the difficulty you will have in quitting.

What Is Nicotine Withdrawal?

Many individuals who stop smoking experience withdrawal symptoms from nicotine. These may include irritability and anger, anxiety, difficulty concentrating, increased appetite and weight gain, and difficulty sleeping. You should be aware that you may experience one or more of these symptoms when you quit smoking.

Many smokers light up a cigarette with their morning coffee, after a meal, and when drinking alcohol. These triggers contribute to the difficulty that some people have when quitting smoking because they associate one activity (smoking) with another (morning coffee). You should be aware of these conditions and have a plan to overcome them. You may wish to avoid such triggers by going for a walk or exercising, talking to a friend, or calling a helpline dedicated to those who are struggling to quit smoking.

What Should I Do If I Want to Quit Smoking?

Start the process by thinking about what you like and do not like about smoking. You may want to actually write these things down on a piece of paper. Then, you should set a quit date and tell your family and friends that you plan to quit smoking. Next, remove cigarettes and other tobacco products from your home, car, and place of work. You should anticipate some tough times while you are quitting and have a plan to deal with these. The plan may need to include talking with your doctor or attending a smoking cessation program. Most programs include behavioral counseling so that a professional can help you examine your smoking triggers, ways to overcome cravings, and what went wrong when you tried to quit before.

Check with your local hospital or medical center to find out what services are offered. You may also want to check out what is offered online or call one of the resources listed in this book. Smoking cessation depends on your desire and commitment to quit. Numerous programs are available to help you. The first step? You must want to quit smoking.

Resources for Smoking Cessation

Organization	Website	Phone
American Lung Association	www.lung.org	800-586-4672
Freedom from Smoking®	www.ffsonline.org	
COPD Foundation	www.copd.foundation.org	866-316-2673
Tobacco Quit Line		800 QUIT NOW
American Cancer Society	www.cancer.org	
Federal Government	www. smokefree.gov	

What Medications Can Help Me Quit Smoking?

Only about 10 percent of people who quit smoking cold turkey are successful. Therefore, you should consider different medications, such as nicotine replacement, bupropion (brand name: Wellbutrin), and varenicline (brand name: Chantix), to help you stop smoking.

With nicotine replacement therapies, the nicotine is absorbed into the blood from gum, lozenges, a skin patch, nasal spray, or an inhaler. The levels of nicotine that reach the blood are generally lower than you would achieve by smoking a pack of cigarettes each day.

Nicotine Replacement Therapies

Available over the counter

Gum contains nicotine at doses of 2 and 4 mg that is slowly released with chewing and is absorbed through the cheek or gums. You should chew the gum until you feel a tingling sensation, and then move the gum under your lip. Park the gum there for two to five minutes while the nicotine is absorbed into your body. Then, repeat the process as long as you want. Use when needed, such as when you crave a cigarette. At the start, you may chew a piece of gum as often as you smoked a cigarette. The 2 mg gum should be chewed if you smoked twenty-five cigarettes or fewer per day. The 4 mg dose is recommended if you smoked more than twenty-five cigarettes per day.

Lozenges slowly release nicotine into saliva, which is then absorbed similar to gum.

Patches allow nicotine to be absorbed through the skin and into the blood. The doses are 7, 14, and 21 mg. The highest dose (21 mg) is usually recommended initially, and the patch should be worn for two to three months.

Prescription required

Nasal spray delivers a liquid solution of nicotine into the nose where it is absorbed into the blood. This may cause some irritation of the nose.

Inhalers release nicotine when you inhale through the device. The nicotine is then absorbed slowly through the mouth similar to gum and lozenges. Irritation of the mouth and throat may occur.

Nicotine replacement therapy eases your body's craving for nicotine and subsequent withdrawal symptoms. The dose of most of these products depends on the number of cigarettes that you smoke each day. The dose is generally tapered as you experience fewer withdrawal symptoms. In general, nicotine replacement therapy is recommended for two to three months. You should discuss the starting dose of the nicotine product and possible side effects with your doctor or a smoking cessation counselor.

Bupropion and varenicline are prescription medications approved to help individuals quit smoking. Bupropion works in the brain to reduce your desire to smoke. This medication is also used to treat depression and seasonal affective disorder. The starting dose is a 150 mg tablet once a day for the first three days, and then twice a day after that. You should take this medication for at least one week before your target quit date. Treatment typically continues for seven to twelve weeks. However, you should not take this medication if you have a history of seizures or an eating disorder such as anorexia or bulimia. You should discuss possible side effects of bupropion with your doctor. The most serious side effects are the risk of suicidal thoughts and depression.

Varenicline is a prescription medication that works in the brain to reduce withdrawal symptoms and cravings for cigarettes. You should take this medication for at least one week before your target quit date. The starting dose is 0.5 mg daily for three days, then twice daily for four days, and then 1 mg twice daily for the remainder of a twelve-week course. You should discuss possible side effects of varenicline with your doctor. The most serious side effects are the risk of suicidal thoughts and possible cardiac events in those with known heart disease. Other possible effects include a higher rate of injuries from driving accidents and falls.

What Is an E-cigarette?

An electronic cigarette, or e-cigarette, consists of a liquid cartridge that contains nicotine, propylene glycol, and other chemicals. A battery powers a heating element that creates a vapor resembling smoke. The dose of nicotine, a highly addictive chemical, varies with the vigor used to inhale. Propylene glycol is an irritant to the lungs, and its long-term safety is unknown. E-cigarettes lack quality control on the dose of nicotine and contain inconsistent contents.

Tobacco companies make e-cigarettes and have generally marketed these products as an alternative to smoking cigarettes as opposed to a solution for those hoping to quit smoking. At the present time, there are concerns about the safety of e-cigarettes and lack of regulatory oversight of the manufacturing process.

What Else Can I Do to Quit Smoking?

Lifestyle changes can help you quit smoking. These include learning relaxation techniques to reduce stress and starting an exercise program to improve your health and fitness. Stay away from family members or friends when they smoke. For example, you can ask a family member to smoke outside rather than in the house. You may also want to deal with cravings by keeping some oral substitutes nearby, such as sugarless gum, carrots, or sunflower seeds. It is important to remember that cravings for a cigarette will slowly subside. Do not think that smoking just one more cigarette won't hurt you. Most of the time, smoking one cigarette leads to smoking more.

It is very important that you have support to help you quit smoking as you transition to becoming a non-smoker. Family and friends will hopefully be at the top of the list to provide support. In addition, a healthcare provider, counselor, or a person at the other end of a telephone hotline may be helpful. You may wish to talk to someone about different temptations that might occur when you quit smoking, possible withdrawal symptoms, and concerns about weight gain.

Group counseling is available at various health organizations and local hospitals, and typically includes lectures on coping skills and group meetings. Some individuals report success using hypnosis or acupuncture. It doesn't matter which method you use to quit smoking as long as the treatment is safe.

Key Points

1. The greatest barrier to quitting smoking is addiction to nicotine.
2. When you stop smoking, you will likely experience withdrawal symptoms, such as irritability, anxiety, difficulty concentrating, increased appetite, and difficulty sleeping. These may be mild or severe, and, though temporary, may last a few weeks.
3. Only 10 percent of people who quit smoking cold turkey are successful. Nicotine replacement therapy, as well as prescription medications such as bupropion or varenicline, can help you quit.
4. You should discuss these medications with your doctor.
5. To help you quit smoking, you may wish to learn relaxation techniques, start an exercise program, ask your family and friends for support and encouragement, attend a stop-smoking program, participate in group counseling, or talk to an expert on a quit-smoking telephone hotline.

Follow-Up Vignette

James discussed his desire to quit smoking with his doctor. The doctor explained how nicotine in cigarette smoke is addictive, and described different treatment options with James. After their discussion, James decided to start the nicotine patch at the 21 mg dose. The doctor congratulated James on his plans to quit smoking and suggested that he attend the stop-smoking program at the local hospital. James and his wife agreed that he would not have any cigarettes at home or in the car starting on his quit date. James told his brother, also a smoker, that he did not want to do things together for a while since James was quitting smoking. His brother said that he understood the situation.

James was successful quitting smoking for three weeks. Then, a grandson was hospitalized with pneumonia. James became upset and worried a lot about his grandson. He decided to stop the nicotine patch, and started smoking again to "calm his nerves." His grandson slowly recovered, was discharged from the hospital, and returned to school a few weeks later.

Several months went by while James continued to smoke a pack of cigarettes per day. James had canceled his follow-up appointment with his doctor when his grandson was sick. James felt guilty and did not want to tell his doctor that he had started smoking again. In addition, James's wife noticed that he had lost interest in gardening, yard work, and fishing. She convinced James to see his doctor again to get help.

At the appointment, James reluctantly explained the situation to his doctor, and acknowledged that he was "feeling down." The doctor recommended that James start bupropion to both help him quit smoking and to treat his depression. James agreed with this plan and expressed interest in attending the stop-smoking program at the local hospital.

James was apprehensive about attending his first stop smoking meeting. However, he realized that everyone else at the meeting was nervous as well. He listened to the group leader and what others had to say about the challenges of not smoking. After a few weeks, James realized that bupropion was helping to take away his desire to smoke, and that he was ready to quit smoking. He threw his cigarettes away, and told his wife that he was finished with smoking. James asked for support and understanding from his family members. One month later, James and his family enjoyed a picnic together to celebrate his success.

CHAPTER 4

Can You Help Me Breathe Easier?

Vignette

Larry is a fifty-seven-year-old man who was diagnosed with COPD two years ago. His family doctor prescribed an inhaler containing albuterol and ipratropium (brand name: Combivent) to use three to four times a day. Larry reported that this medication was helpful, but lasted only about four hours, and then he would be short of breath when doing activities like raking leaves or bending down to paint. Over the past year, he would wake up in the middle of the night about once a week because he "couldn't catch his breath." He used the inhaler, which helped. Larry and his wife decided to ask his doctor what else could be done to help him breathe.

Introduction

The following strategies are simple and inexpensive and can provide some relief for your breathlessness.

Pursed-lips breathing

Exhaling through pursed lips can be used when you experience distress or difficulty breathing. The following instructions and illustrations demonstrate this breathing technique.

Start by sitting in a comfortable position and relax.

A. Take a slow, deep breath in through your nose.
B. Purse or pucker your lips together as if you were going to whistle.

C. Breathe out slowly through your mouth and empty the air from your lungs.

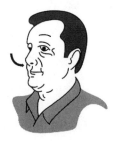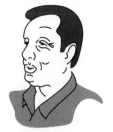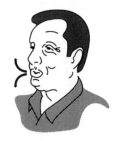

FIGURE 12

A. Inhale through nose   B. Purse or pucker lips   C. Exhale through mouth

Studies have shown that pursed-lips breathing can increase the level of oxygen in the blood and will decrease breathing frequency. In addition, many individuals with COPD describe a sense of breathing control when exhaling through pursed lips. You should try this breathing technique when your breathing is stable in order to practice the three steps.

Forward-leaning position

Some people with COPD experience marked relief of breathing difficulty when leaning forward with hands and forearms positioned on the thighs or supported by a table or shopping cart. The forward-leaning position enables the neck and rib muscles to assist the —the diaphragm muscle— to breathe in.

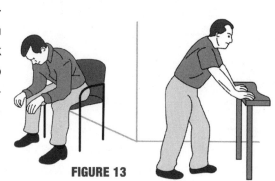

FIGURE 13

Fans

Many individuals with COPD report that movement of cool air, especially when seated near an open window or in front of a fan, eases their breathing. The benefit of air movement is likely due to activation of sensors on the face that send signals to the brain. Options include sitting a few feet from a pedestal fan or holding a small portable battery-operated fan in one hand with airflow directed toward the face.

Music

Listening to music can be enjoyable and relaxing. Depending on the type, many people find music to be a pleasant distraction. In a study involving those with COPD, listening to music while walking improved performance and reduced breathlessness compared to another group of people with COPD who also walked but did not listen to music.[6] It is possible that the benefits of music for relieving breathing discomfort may be tied to its relaxing effect on the brain. It is reasonable for someone who has COPD to listen to his or her favorite music to assess whether this activity might be helpful. At the very least, music may distract you from thinking about your trouble breathing.

Endorphins

Endorphins are naturally-occurring narcotic substances similar to morphine that are produced in the brain. They are released into the fluid around the brain and into the blood when you exercise for a period of time, when you have surgery, when you experience pain, and when you have severe breathing difficulty. Studies show that endorphins relieve breathing difficulty in those with COPD.[7, 8] It is possible, but not proven, that certain activities that promote the release of endorphins may improve your breathing discomfort. You may want to try one or more of these and note whether these activities help your shortness of breath.

Activities that Release Endorphins

Exercise
Laughing
Eating chocolate or hot peppers
Drinking liquids containing caffeine

What Medicines Are Available to Relieve My Breathing Difficulty?

Various medications have been approved by the Food and Drug Administration (FDA) and similar agencies throughout the world for the treatment of COPD. One type of medication is called a bronchodilator, which increases airflow by relaxing the muscle that wraps around the airways (see Chapter 1). Another type of medication is called a corticosteroid, which reduces redness and inflammation in the airway. An inhaled corticosteroid has been approved by the FDA only when used together with a specific type of bronchodilator called a beta-agonist. The separate effects of these two types of inhaled medications are summarized and illustrated below.

Two Types of Inhaled Medications Used to Treat COPD

Bronchodilators → Relax bronchial smooth muscle
Corticosteroids → Reduce airway inflammation

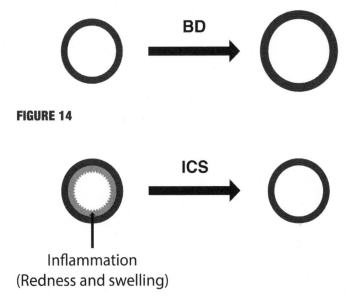

FIGURE 14

Inflammation
(Redness and swelling)

These figures show the size of airways as viewed by looking straight through the breathing tubes. The diameter of the airway increases as a result of inhaling a bronchodilator (BD), which relaxes bronchial smooth muscle. At the bottom left, the inner irregular circle represents inflammation inside the airway. The internal diameter of the airway increases as a result of inhaling a corticosteroid (ICS), which reduces airway inflammation.

By improving airflow, these types of medications allow more air to be exhaled, which deflates the lungs, like letting air out of a balloon. The beneficial effects of deflation are shown in Figure 15. The primary effect is that the diaphragm muscle is able to work more efficiently. Increased airflow and deflation of the lungs are the main reasons that these medications make it easier for you to breathe.

Daily use of long-acting bronchodilators will allow you to gain even greater benefits when combined with participation in a pulmonary rehabilitation program (see Chapter 7).

Deflation of the Lungs

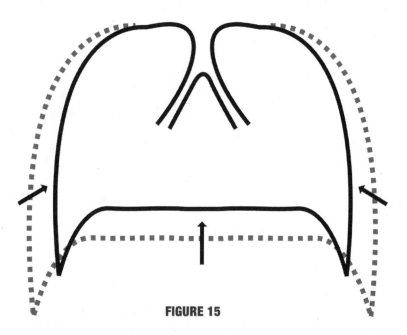

FIGURE 15

An increase in airflow enables the diaphragm to move up (upward arrow) and the chest wall to move inward (diagonal arrows). This better empties the lungs, allowing the diaphragm to function more efficiently.

Why Are There Different Types of Bronchodilators?

There are two different types, or classes, of bronchodilators based on how the medications act on bronchial smooth muscle. One type is called a beta-agonist, and the other type is called a muscarinic antagonist. A simple explanation is illustrated below.

Types of Bronchodilators	
Class	**Mechanism**
Beta-agonist	Increases a chemical that relaxes smooth muscle
Muscarinic antagonist	Blocks a receptor in smooth muscle

Ω Airflow

Why is this important to you? Because these two different types of inhaled bronchodilators work in different ways to improve airflow and deflate the lungs. Using a beta-agonist and a muscarinic antagonist in combination works better than using only one of these bronchodilators alone.

What Are the Beta-agonist Bronchodilators?

These medications are similar to adrenaline (also known as epinephrine) and are classified by how many hours they keep the airways open. It is important that you know either the brand or generic name of the beta-agonist bronchodilator that you are using and how long it is expected to last. If this information is hard to remember, you should have this information written down and bring this with you to your next doctor's appointment.

Why is this important to you? Because the number of hours that the medication works determines how often you should take it. The following tables list the names of the medications, whether the medication is an aerosol, dry powder, or liquid solution, and how many hours the medication is expected to work. An aerosol is delivered by a metered-dose inhaler commonly called a puffer. A dry powder is delivered by a dry-powder inhaler, and a solution is delivered in a nebulizer.

Commonly Used Beta-agonist Bronchodilators

Short-acting (last 4-6 hours)

Generic Name	Brand name™	Substance
Albuterol sulfate	Pro-Air	aerosol
	Proventil	aerosol
	Ventolin	aerosol
Albuterol sulfate		solution
Levalbuterol tartrate	Xopenex	aerosol and solution

Long-acting (last 12 hours)

Generic Name	Brand name™	Substance
Arformoterol tartrate	Brovana	solution
Formoterol fumarate	Perforomist	solution
Formoterol fumarate	Foradil Aerolizer	dry powder
Salmeterol xinafoate	Serevent Diskus	dry powder

Long-acting once daily (last 24 hours)

Generic Name	Brand name™	Substance
Indacaterol	Arcapta Neohaler	dry powder
Olodaterol	Striverdi Respimat	soft mist

™ The brands are registered trademarks of specific pharmaceutical companies

All of the beta-agonists listed in the table, except for salmeterol, start working in five minutes to open your airways. You may or may not notice an improvement in your breathing this quickly. In general, a short-acting beta-agonist (albuterol) should be used as needed. This means that you should inhale one or two puffs of albuterol when you experience breathing difficulty, or before doing an activity that you expect will cause you to become breathless, such as walking or going to the store. In contrast, long-acting beta-agonists are used as maintenance therapy.

Rescue Use

- Short-acting: Can be used every four hours as needed.

Maintenance or Regular Use

- Long-acting (lasts up to twelve hours): Can be taken twice a day about twelve hours apart.
- Long-acting once daily: Used once a day in the morning.

You should be aware that in 2005 the FDA issued a warning that long-acting beta-agonists "increase the risk of asthma-related death." However, long-acting beta-agonists are considered safe and are used routinely to treat those with COPD. In a three-year study involving over 6,000 patients with COPD, salmeterol, a long-acting beta-agonist used twice daily, was as safe as a placebo.[9]

The following information describes possible side effects of beta-agonists. If you have concerns, or if you have experienced any of these possible side effects, you should talk with your doctor.

Possible Side Effects of Beta-agonists

Mild: shakiness (tremor); nervousness; anxiety; trouble sleeping; increased heart rate

Serious: irregular or very fast heart rate; seizures; low potassium in blood

What Are the Muscarinic Antagonist Bronchodilators?

A muscarinic antagonist blocks a receptor in bronchial smooth muscle that causes constriction. Blocking this receptor enables the muscle around the airways to relax. Like beta-agonists, these bronchodilators are classified by how long they keep the airways open. Once again, it is important that you know the generic or brand name of the muscarinic antagonist bronchodilator that you are taking and how long it is expected to last.

Commonly Used Muscarinic Antagonist Bronchodilators

Short-acting (last 4-6 hours)

Generic Name	Brand name™	Substance
Ipratropium bromide	Atrovent HFA	aerosol and solution

Long-acting (last 12 hours)

Generic Name	Brand name™	Substance
Aclidinium bromide	Tudorza Pressair	dry powder

Long-acting once daily (last 24 hours)

Generic Name	Brand name™	Substance
Tiotropium	Spiriva HandiHaler	dry powder
Umeclidinium	Incruse Ellipta	dry powder

™ The brands are registered trademarks of specific pharmaceutical companies

Muscarinic antagonists do *not* act quickly to open your airways, and have a peak effect at about two hours after inhalation. This means that this class of bronchodilator is used as maintenance four times a day (ipratropium bromide), twice a day (aclinidium bromide), or once a day (tiotropium and umeclidinium). Muscarinic antagonists are considered safe and are used routinely by those with COPD. In a three-year study involving over 6,000 patients with COPD, tiotropium was as safe as a placebo.[10]

The following information describes possible side effects of muscarinic antagonists. If you have concerns, or if you have any of these symptoms, talk with your doctor.

Possible Side Effects of Muscarinic Antagonists

Mild: dryness of the mouth; cough; headache

Serious: difficulty urinating, especially in older men; glaucoma

Are There Combination Medications for COPD?

Several inhaled combination medications are available, and these offer two advantages. First, the use of two medications is typically more effective than using either one alone. Second, it is convenient to use a single inhaler rather than two separate inhalers. For the treatment of COPD, the FDA has approved combining two bronchodilators (a beta-agonist and a muscarinic antagonist) and combining an inhaled corticosteroid with a long-acting beta-agonist. The combination of two different types of bronchodilators offers the advantage of greater improvement in breathing difficulty compared with only one bronchodilator.

Combination of Two Bronchodilator Medications		
Short-acting (last 4-6 hours)		
Generic Name	**Brand name™**	**Substance**
Albuterol sulfate and	Combivent Respimat	soft mist
ipratropium bromide	DuoNeb	solution

Combination of Two Bronchodilator Medications

Long-acting once daily (last 24 hours)

Generic Name	Brand name™	Substance
Umeclidinium and vilanterol	Anoro Ellipta	dry powder

™ The brands are registered trademarks of specific pharmaceutical companies

Another combination medication includes an inhaled corticosteroid with a beta-agonist bronchodilator. These two medications work by reducing inflammation and by relaxing bronchial smooth muscle. One specific benefit of this type of combination medication is reducing exacerbations, which are episodes of increased breathing difficulty usually due to a chest infection, among patients with severe COPD and with a history of exacerbations (see Chapter 8).

Combination of Inhaled Corticosteroid and Beta-agonist Bronchodilator

Long-acting (last 12 hours)

Generic Name	Brand name™	Substance
Fluticasone propionate and salmeterol	Advair Diskus	dry powder
	Advair HFA	aerosol
Budesonide and formoterol fumarate	Symbicort	aerosol

Long-acting once daily (last 24 hours)

Generic Name	Brand name™	Substance
Fluticasone furoate and vilanterol	Breo Ellipta	dry powder

™ The brands are registered trademarks of specific pharmaceutical companies

Both types of combination medications are used widely and are generally safe. Possible side effects of beta-agonists and muscarinic antagonists are listed on the previous pages. Inhaled corticosteroids may cause hoarseness, oral candidiasis (a yeast infection in the throat), bruising of the skin, osteoporosis, and an increase in the risk of pneumonia. You should rinse your mouth with water after using an inhaled corticosteroid and beta-agonist combination to prevent a yeast infection. Make sure to discuss any concerns that you may have about combination medications with your doctor.

Possible Side Effects of Inhaled Corticosteroids

Mild: hoarseness; yeast infection in throat; bruising of skin

Serious: cataracts; osteoporosis; pneumonia

Are There Pills that Can Help Me Breathe Easier?

Theophylline is a pill that is similar to caffeine. In the past, theophylline was used frequently to treat those with COPD. Like other bronchodilators, theophylline relaxes bronchial smooth muscle and deflates the lung. At the present time, theophylline is not used widely, but may be tried for those individuals who continue to experience breathing difficulty despite use of both types of bronchodilators and an inhaled corticosteroid. Use of these three inhaled medications is called triple therapy.

Theophylline should not be used if you have heart disease because it may cause an irregular heart rhythm. The following information lists possible side effects of theophylline.

Possible Side Effects of Theophylline

Mild: shakiness (tremor); nervousness; anxiety; trouble sleeping; increased heart rate; nausea; upset stomach; headache

Serious: irregular or very fast heart rate; seizures

If you experience any of these problems and are taking theophylline, you should talk to your doctor immediately. As theophylline may interact with other medications, make sure to tell your physician about all prescription and over-the-counter medications that you are taking.

Key Points

1. Try pursed-lips breathing, the forward-leaning position, the use of a fan, and listening to music to help ease your breathing difficulty.
2. If your breathing problem limits your daily activities, tell your doctor and ask what treatments are available.
3. It is important to know the names of all medications that you are using for COPD. Write this information down on paper or enter it into your laptop or smartphone and take this information with you to your doctor's appointment.
4. You should understand the different types of medications that are available to help your breathing.
5. Long-acting bronchodilators are more effective than short-acting bronchodilators. These are available to use either once or twice a day.

Follow-Up Vignette

Larry discussed his shortness of breath with his doctor, and asked what else was available to help his breathing problem. The doctor informed Larry about simple measures to try at home, including pursed-lips breathing, the forward-leaning position, use of a fan, and listening to music.

The doctor also discussed the different types of once- or twice-daily bronchodilators that were available. The doctor presented Larry with two possible options:

- start a once-daily bronchodilator (beta-agonist or muscarinic antagonist) in the morning, and return for a follow-up visit in a few weeks to assess its effect; or
- start a combination beta-agonist and muscarinic antagonist in a single inhaler

After discussing medications with his doctor, Larry chose the second option—the dual bronchodilator combination. Since the two different bronchodilators would work in different ways to open up the airways, Larry was hopeful that he would achieve greater relief in his breathing difficulty.

CHAPTER 5

How Should I Use My Inhalers?

Vignette

J anet was diagnosed with COPD a few months ago at age fifty-seven. An albuterol inhaler and a dry-powder bronchodilator were prescribed. Janet tried both medications, but found that neither one helped her breathe easier. She recently moved to be near one of her children, and had lots of breathing problems while packing, carrying boxes, and unpacking. She made an appointment with a doctor in her new location to ask what other medications she could use.

At her appointment, the doctor asked how she was using the two different inhalers. Janet commented that no one had actually showed her how to properly use the inhalers. The doctor said the nurse would review with her how to inhale the albuterol and dry-powder medications.

Introduction

Inhaled bronchodilators are the preferred method for delivery of medications to treat COPD. The medication is inhaled into the mouth, passes through the throat and between the vocal cords, and then enters the trachea, or windpipe, before reaching the lower airways. The ability of an individual to inhale a medication deep into the lungs depends on correct technique, including having enough force to breathe in. The major advantage of inhaling a medication is that it acts directly in airways of the lungs with minimal effect on other parts of the body. This approach reduces possible side effects compared with swallowing a pill.

What Are the Different Devices for Inhaling Medications?

As noted in Chapter 4, inhaled bronchodilators relax the muscle around the airways, while inhaled corticosteroids reduce inflammation inside the airways. There are three major delivery systems:

- aerosol (spray) in a metered-dose inhaler (MDI)
- powder in a dry-powder inhaler (DPI)
- solution in a nebulizer machine

It is important for you to understand these delivery systems in order to achieve the greatest benefit. The following information describes why different inhaling techniques are required with each type of medication. Remember, you need to be able to inhale the medication deep into the airways in order for the medicine to work.

How Should I Use an MDI?

An MDI is a handheld aerosol device that releases a specific amount of water droplets mixed with air. The MDI is a pressurized canister inside a plastic holder with a mouthpiece attached at one end. When the canister is pushed down, or activated, the aerosol medication is released. Even with correct inhalation technique, only about 10 percent of what comes out of the inhaler actually reaches the lower airways.

The following instructions describe the open-mouth inhalation technique for using an MDI. You should review each step before using your MDI medication to make sure that you are inhaling properly. If you do not follow the instructions correctly, even less of the medication will reach your lungs. You might also consider asking your doctor or nurse to watch you when you inhale medication from the MDI to confirm that you are doing so properly.

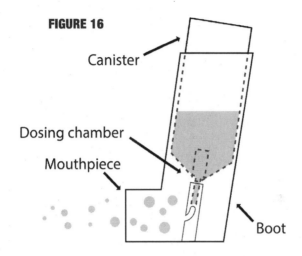

FIGURE 16

Canister

Dosing chamber

Mouthpiece

Boot

Instructions for Using a Metered-Dose Inhaler

1. Shake the MDI vigorously for five seconds.
2. Take the cap off of the mouthpiece.
3. Hold the MDI upright with your index finger on top of the canister and your thumb at the bottom of the inhaler.
4. Breathe out normally.
5. Place the MDI one to two fingers in front of your mouth; this is called the open-mouth technique.
6. As you start to breathe in slowly through your mouth, press down on the top of the canister with your index finger to release the medication.
7. Keep breathing in with a slow and steady force until you fill your lungs with air.
8. Hold your breath for ten seconds or as long as possible. This allows the aerosol to reach the lower airways.
9. Wait fifteen to thirty seconds, and then take a second puff.
10. If the medication contains an inhaled corticosteroid, you should rinse your mouth with water and spit the water out.

If your MDI is new, or if it has not been used in two weeks, you need to prime the inhaler as described below. Priming enables you to get the full dose of the inhaled medication. Each pharmaceutical company provides recommendations for priming the particular MDI.

Priming Your Metered-Dose Inhaler

1. Shake the MDI vigorously for five seconds.
2. Take the cap off of the mouthpiece.
3. Press down on the canister and spray the aerosol away from you three to four times into the air. This will waste three to four puffs.
4. The MDI is now ready for use.

Should I Use a Spacer with my MDI?

Appropriate use of an MDI requires coordination between your finger pressing down on the canister and breathing in. A spacer device may be recommended to use with the MDI if you have difficulty with coordination or if you are using an MDI that contains an inhaled corticosteroid. A spacer is shown in Figure 17 and serves as a reservoir for the medication from the MDI. You should ask your doctor whether a spacer is necessary.

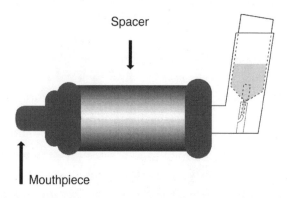

Spacer

Mouthpiece

FIGURE 17. Example of a spacer with a metered-dose inhaler.

The spacer holds the aerosol medication long enough for you to inhale slow and steady. You shold *not* exhale into the spacer, as that will dilute the available medication to be inhaled. A spacer will also decrease the amount of aerosol deposited in the mouth and throat.

Instructions for Using an MDI with a Spacer

1. Shake the MDI vigorously for five seconds.
2. Take the cap off of the mouthpiece.
3. Place the MDI into the end of the spacer.
4. Breathe out normally away from the spacer.
5. Put your mouth around the mouthpiece of the spacer and close your lips.
6. Press down on the top of the MDI canister with your index finger to release the medication into the spacer.
7. Breathe in very slowly until you have filled your lungs with air.
8. If you hear a whistle sound, you are breathing in too fast.
9. Hold your breath for ten seconds or as long as possible. This allows the aerosol to reach the lower airways.
10. Wait fifteen to thirty seconds and then repeat for the second puff.
11. If the medication contains an inhaled corticosteroid, rinse your mouth with water and spit the water out.

How Should I Use the Respimat Inhaler?

The Respimat inhaler is unique in that it delivers a soft mist through a nozzle. The instructions for using this device are slightly different than the instructions for using an MDI. First, turn the clear base in the direction of the arrows. You will hear a click. Then, open the cap. You should breathe out slowly, and then place your lips around the end of the mouthpiece. Then, while taking a slow and deep breath in, press the dose-release button and continue to breathe in slowly for as long as possible. Then, hold your breath for ten seconds or as long as possible. You may want to ask your doctor or nurse to observe you inhaling from this inhaler.

How Should I Use a DPI?

A DPI is a device that contains a dry-powder medication inhaled into the lungs. The medication is either stored in powder packets inside the device or held in a capsule to be loaded into the device with each use. The force of your inhalation breaks up the powder into small particles that can reach the lower airways.

A DPI is breath-actuated, which means that no coordination is required between activating the device and inhaling the medication. Each DPI has an internal resistance, which means you need to breathe in hard and fast to break up the powder into little particles. This requires that you have an adequate force when breathing in. If you do not breathe in hard and fast and hold your breath for ten seconds, or for as long as possible, a lot of the medication will be deposited in your mouth and throat. You should discuss the correct inhalation technique with your doctor or nurse; each DPI has slightly different instructions for use.

What If the DPI Isn't Helping Me Breathe Easier?

If you are not sure whether the dry-powder medication is helping your breathing, talk to your doctor. Your doctor may wish to measure your peak inspiratory flow rate (PIFR). This is a simple breathing test that measures your force of breathing in.

A low value for PIFR (usually less than 60 liters/minute) indicates that you may not have enough force to inhale the powder deep into the airways. In one study, about one in five patients, or 20 percent, who were at least sixty years of age

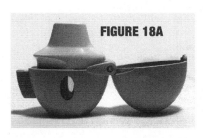

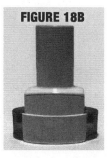

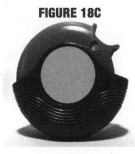

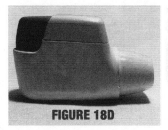

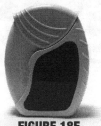

Examples of single-dose (Figures a and b) and multiple-dose (Figures c, d, and e) dry-powder inhalers. a = HandiHaler; b = Neohaler; c = Diskus; d = Pressair; e = Ellipta

with severe COPD had a PIFR below 60 liters/minute when inhaling against a resistance similar to the Diskus.[11]

Why is this important? If your inspiratory flow rate is low, you may not be able to inhale the dry-powder medication deep into the airways. If that is the case, then it is unlikely that the medication will help your breathing. Your doctor may decide to prescribe medications that can be inhaled from a nebulizer machine.

How Should I Use a Nebulizer?

Another approach is to inhale a solution placed into a neb-ulizer machine. Nebulizers use oxygen, compressed air, or ultrasonic power to break up a liquid medication into a mist that can be inhaled from a mouthpiece connected to the nebulizer. There are portable nebulizers with the option of a rechargeable battery that you can take with you when you travel. A car adapter may also be used to power the device.

Nebulizer

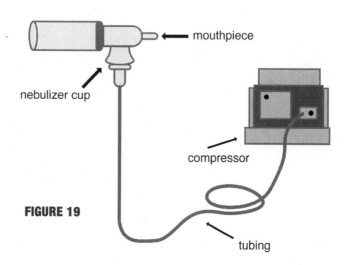

mouthpiece

nebulizer cup

compressor

FIGURE 19

tubing

Example of a nebulizer.

Inhaling a medication from a nebulizer is recommended if you:

- are unable to use the MDI or DPI because of a physical problem, such as arthritis or a stroke
- have difficulty coordinating your breathing and holding your breath
- do not find it easier to breathe with the MDI or DPI despite using correct technique
- have a low PIFR

A nebulizer machine and the associated medications can be ordered by your doctor. A person who works for a home care company, usually a nurse or respiratory therapist, typically delivers both the nebulizer and medications to you at home and will instruct you how to set up and clean the system. The nebulizer and medications may also be obtained at a pharmacy. The following information describes how to inhale the medication from a nebulizer.

Instructions for Using a Nebulizer

1. Wash your hands with soap and water.
2. Place the nebulizer on a hard surface and make sure that the air filter is clean.
3. Open the medication vial and place the solution into the nebulizer container; this may also be called a cup.
4. Make sure that the medication container is connected to the nebulizer.
5. Place the mouthpiece into your mouth and close your lips.
6. Turn on the nebulizer.
7. Breathe in and out normally.
8. Continue until the solution is gone; the nebulizer may begin to sputter.
9. After each use, clean the medication container with mild soap and water and allow to air-dry.
10. Follow any other directions from the manufacturer for cleaning the nebulizer system.

Many individuals with COPD report that nebulized medications are more helpful in improving their breathing. One possible reason is that the dose of the medication used in a nebulizer is considerably higher than the dose of the same medication available in an inhaler. You may experience more side effects with a nebulized medication as a result of the higher dose. These side effects may include shakiness, tremor, and rapid heart rate. You should discuss any concerns or questions with your doctor.

Key Points

1. Different types of inhalers require different breathing techniques.

Recommended Inhalation Techniques

Inhaler	Type of Inhalation
Metered-dose inhaler	slow and steady
MDI with spacer	slow and steady
Respimat inhaler	slow and steady
Dry-powder inhaler	hard and fast
Solution in nebulizer	normal breathing in and out

2. With an MDI (with or without a spacer), Respimat inhaler, and DPI, you should hold your breath as long as possible. With a nebulizer, there is no need to hold your breath.
3. You should consider whether each inhaler medication is helping you breathe easier. If the medication does not help, tell your doctor.
4. Ask your doctor or a nurse to watch you inhale the different medications to make sure that you are doing so correctly.

Follow-Up Vignette

The nurse reviewed with Janet how to inhale from the albuterol MDI and the DPI, and explained that each inhaler worked in a different way. She instructed Janet to use the open-mouth technique with her MDI, using a slow, steady inhalation and holding her breath "for as long as possible." The nurse also showed Janet a DPI and explained that she should inhale "hard and fast" in order to overcome the resistance of the device and break up the powder into tiny particles.

The nurse observed Janet inhaling the different medications from the MDI and DPI, and congratulated her on "doing it right." Finally, the nurse gave Janet written instructions that illustrated how to inhale correctly with the MDI and DPI.

At a follow-up visit one month later, Janet informed both the doctor and the nurse that the medications were helping her breathe easier since she was now using them correctly.

CHAPTER 6

Do I Need Oxygen?

Vignette

Clifford, a seventy-six-year-old man with severe COPD, was recently admitted to the hospital for a chest infection that caused his breathing to worsen. Oxygen was prescribed for Clifford in the hospital, and he was discharged home with instructions to use oxygen 24/7. He was worried that he might need oxygen for the rest of his life.

At the visit with his doctor two weeks later, Clifford reported that he was feeling better, and wanted to know if he needed to use oxygen "all of the time." He had stopped using oxygen for up to thirty minutes while reading the newspaper and watching television, and felt that his breathing was fine. However, Clifford's wife was nervous when he stopped using oxygen, and wanted him to ask the doctor whether doing so was safe.

Introduction

Everybody knows that oxygen is required for our bodies to function. The air that we breathe contains 21 percent oxygen. Normally, oxygen is inhaled into the airways, reaches the air sacs, and goes into the blood. Red blood cells carry oxygen to all parts of the body where it is used by cells to produce energy and to perform specific functions. In some individuals with COPD, destruction in the lungs reduces the ability of oxygen to enter the blood. This results in lower-than-normal levels of oxygen in the body.

How Is My Oxygen Level Measured?

A pulse oximeter is placed on a finger to measure the amount of oxygen bound to red blood cells. The measurement is simple and noninvasive. An oximeter works by passing two different wavelengths of light through the finger, and a sensor on the opposite side detects the amount of oxygen in the blood. A pulse oximeter provides two numbers:

- oxygen saturation, abbreviated by SpO_2, is a percentage where S = saturation, p = pulse, and O_2 = oxygen
- heart rate is measured as beats per minute

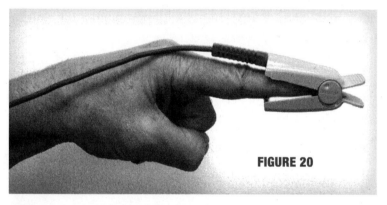

FIGURE 20

Side view of pulse oximeter positioned on a finger.

The accuracy of the oximeter depends on the sensor detecting each pulse, or flow of blood, in the finger coming from the heart. If there is poor blood flow to the finger, the SpO_2 may provide a false value. This can occur if the hand is cold, if there is a movement of the hand, such as shaking or a tremor, or if the heart is beating irregularly as occurs with atrial fibrillation.

Your doctor may want to measure your oxygen level directly from a blood sample. This test is called an arterial blood gas, abbreviated as ABG. The blood sample also measures your carbon dioxide level, a waste product of our body, and pH, a measure of acid in the blood.

What Is a Normal Oxygen Level?

A normal oxygen saturation level is 95 to 100 percent. These numbers indicate that the air sacs and blood vessels in the lungs are working normally.

How Do I Know If I Need Oxygen?

A low oxygen level is required by insurance companies and Medicare/Medicaid to pay for oyygen therapy. Different conditions determine whether someone qualifies for oxygen.[12] The following information is presented to help you understand whether you qualify for using oxygen at rest, with activities, and/or during sleep.

At Rest

- SpO_2 equal to or less than 88 percent; or
- SpO_2 equal to or less than 89 percent if there is enlargement of the right side of the heart, failure of the right heart, or a high red blood cell level

During Sleep

- SpO_2 equal to or less than 88 percent; or
- there is a fall in SpO_2 of greater than 5 percent with evidence of restlessness, difficulty sleeping, or impaired thinking

During Exercise

- SpO_2 equal to or less than 88 percent; or
- if the person has shortness of breath and high levels of breathing during exercise and the use of oxygen allows the person to increase exercise endurance

You should discuss any questions and concerns about whether you qualify for oxygen with your doctor. If you qualify for oxygen at rest, then you should also use oxygen during sleep and during exercise. This means using it "all of the time." Some individuals may have an SpO_2 value of 89 percent or higher at rest, and therefore do not need to use oxygen when inactive, such as while reading the paper or watching television. However, you may still need to use oxygen if the SpO_2 is 88 percent or lower when you are doing activities and/or during sleep.

Will Oxygen Help Me?

Research studies have shown that if you qualify to use oxygen at rest, using oxygen will help you live longer. Oxygen can also improve your quality of life, make it easier to breathe, and enable you to perform physical activities for a longer stretch of time.[13]

What Are the Available Oxygen Systems?

Oxygen is provided by a stationary or portable sysem. From a machine or tank, oxygen passes through tubing to the nose and/or mouth, and is then inhaled. Your doctor will order an oxygen delivery system along with tubing from a local company, and must sign a certificate that oxygen is medically necessary based on test results. The certificate will indicate whether oxygen should be used at rest, with activities, and/or during sleep, as well as how much oxygen should be given. All equipment will be delivered to your home. The following information describes the different oxygen systems.

Stationary Systems

Oxygen concentrator

This system concentrates oxygen from the air we breathe by removing nitrogen gas. An oxygen concentrator is frequntly used in the home, requires electricity, and should have periodic checkups with filter changes.

Compressed gas in a cyclinder

Oxygen is compressed into a metal cyclinder, or tank, under high pressure. The cyclinder may be small or large and should be secured to prevent it from falling over.

Liquid oxygen

Liquid oxygen can be stored in a large or small tank and is filled by an oxygen supply company usually twice a month. The large tank can be used to fill a small portable tank with liquid oxygen.

In general, portable systems are intended to be used while performing activities, especially outside of the person's home. They are generally small and lightweight (less than ten pounds), and can be used with continuous flow or with a pulse system in which the flow of oxygen occurs only when you breathe in. A pulse system conserves oxygen use and increases the length of time that you can be away from a stationary system. The following information describes the different portable systems that are available.

Portable or Ambulatory Systems

Oxygen concentrator

Portable concentrators can be carried or pulled on wheels. They are powered by battery or by an electrical connection.

FIGURE 21

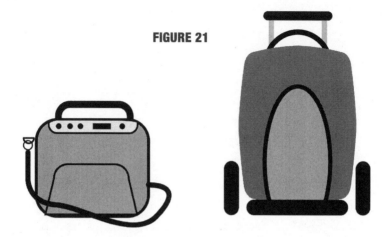

Figure on left is a portable oxygen system that can be carried. Figure on right is a similar system that can be pulled on wheels.

Compressed gas in a cyclinder

Different sizes of compressed gas cyclinders, or tanks, are available. One example is the portable E tank shown in Figure 22. This system is 29 inches in height, weighs 7.9 pounds, and is usually placed on a cart with wheels. It is not particularly easy to use when doing activities, but is good as a backup for stationary concentrators if you lose electrical power. Smaller cyclinders (D tank: 20 inches high and 5.3 pounds; M6 tank: 15 inches high and 2.8 pounds) are available that can be carried over the shoulder or placed in a backpack. Remember, with a smaller cyclinder, the oxygen will run out quicker.

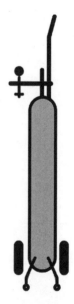

FIGURE 22

Example of a portable E tank.

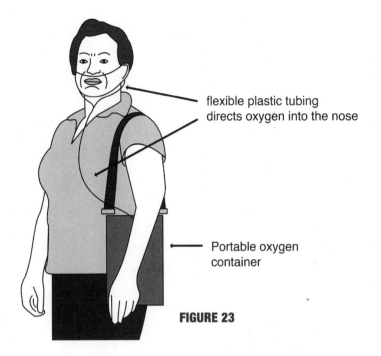

flexible plastic tubing
directs oxygen into the nose

Portable oxygen
container

FIGURE 23

Liquid oxygen

Portable liquid units are filled from a large tank in the home and are available in different sizes.

How Do I Use Oxygen?

Oxygen is delivered through plastic tubing connected to two soft plastic prongs placed in front of each nostril. The oxygen flows to the back of the throat, is mixed with room air, and is then inhaled into the airways until it reaches the air sacs. The amount of oxygen given is measured by a flow rate, which is usually 1–4 liters per minute. If a higher flow rate is required, then oxygen is typically delivered through a mask. A mask is more likely to be used in the hospital or emergency department.

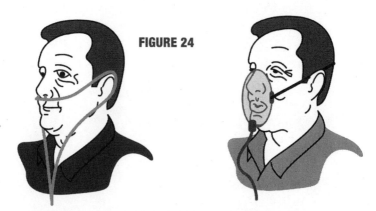

FIGURE 24

Shown on the left is tubing with plastic prongs in each nostril. On the right is a plastic mask over the nose and mouth, which is secured by an elastic strap around the back of the head.

How Much Oxygen Should I Use?

Your physician will determine how much oxygen you should use. The usual goal is to aim for an SpO_2 between 90–92 percent. In most cases, your doctor will request that a nurse, respiratory therapist, or pulmonary function technician adjust the oxygen flow rate while monitoring your SpO_2 with the pulse oximeter at rest and/or when you walk. This is called oxygen titration and determines how much oxygen you should use.

Typically, a higher oxygen flow rate is needed during physical activities than is used at rest. Your doctor may request that your oxygen saturation be measured during sleep to determine if oxygen is required and, if so, an appropriate oxygen flow rate.

Are There Side Effects from Breathing in Oxygen?

Some individuals who use oxygen report that their nose feels dry, and there may be a tendency for a bloody nose. If long tubing is used to deliver oxygen from the concentrator or tank, avoid tripping on the tubing. Certainly, you should not smoke when using oxygen.

Key Points

1. A pulse oximeter can be placed on your finger to measure the amount of oxygen in your blood. The value is called oxygen saturation.
2. A normal oxygen saturation level is 95 percent or higher.
3. Oxygen is recommended if your oxygen saturation level is 88 percent or below.
4. A nurse, respiratory therapist, or pulmonary function technician will use a pulse oximeter to determine how much oxygen you should use at rest, with activities, and/or during sleep.
5. Oxygen is provided by stationary and portable systems.
6. Your doctor will order an oxygen delivery system along with tubing, and will indicate a specific flow rate.
7. Using oxygen should help you breathe easier, improve your quality of life, and increase your ability to be more active.

Follow-Up Vignette

At the clinic visit, the doctor asked Clifford how he was feeling when not using oxygen. The doctor had Clifford turn off the oxygen delivery system in the office because he wanted to measure his oxygen level. For the next fifteen minutes, the doctor continued to ask Clifford questions about his breathing and activity level. The doctor then measured Clifford's oxygen saturation at 92 percent while breathing room air. Next, the doctor asked Clifford to walk in the hallway, and found that the SpO_2 dropped to 85 percent during the brief walk; Clifford said he was starting to feel short of breath. The nurse went to get the portable oxygen system that Clifford had brought with him to the appointment, and had Clifford breathe oxygen at 2 liters/minute. After about ten minutes, his SpO_2 increased to 95 percent at rest. Clifford then walked again in the hallway while breathing oxygen, and his SpO_2 was at 91 percent after walking for two minutes.

The doctor informed Clifford that he did not need to use oxygen at rest, since his SpO_2 was okay at 92 percent, but that he should continue to use oxygen at 2 liters/minute with activities, since his oxygen level had dropped to 85 percent while walking without using oxygen.

Clifford asked about using oxygen when he slept. The doctor told Clifford that the only way to know would be to measure his oxygen saturation when he was sleeping and not using oxygen. The doctor gave Clifford a pulse oximeter to take home so that Clifford could record his SpO_2 levels at night. The oximeter had a computer chip inside to record SpO_2 throughout the night. Clifford was told to bring the machine back the next morning, and that the SpO_2 numbers would indicate whether Clifford would need to use oxygen during sleep.

Both Clifford and his wife were satisfied with the doctor's explanation and the plan to assess the need for oxygen during sleep.

CHAPTER 7

Will Pulmonary Rehabilitation Help Me?

Vignette

Alice is a fifty-nine-year-old woman who noticed that her breathing was getting worse over the past year, especially when shopping at the grocery store and walking fast to catch the bus. She had smoked one pack of cigarettes per day for forty years, but quit smoking one year ago. She had pulmonary function tests six months ago and was told by her doctor that she had "moderate COPD." She and her husband both noted that she was "slowing down." Alice was also aware that she had gained eight pounds over the past few months, which included the Thanksgiving and Christmas holidays.

Alice's sister-in-law had told her about a neighbor who completed the pulmonary rehabilitation program at the local hospital, and he was now able to do yard work again. Alice asked her doctor whether pulmonary rehabilitation would benefit her.

Introduction

Almost everyone who has COPD experiences breathing difficulty (see Chapter 2). When it becomes "hard to breathe" during certain activities, many individuals reduce or stop these activities in order to avoid the unpleasant experience. You may not be aware that you have adjusted your lifestyle, or might blame it on "getting older." Reduced physical activity leads to deconditioning, a word that means being out of shape. When deconditioning occurs, individuals commonly gain weight. This process creates a downward spiral as illustrated in Figure 25.

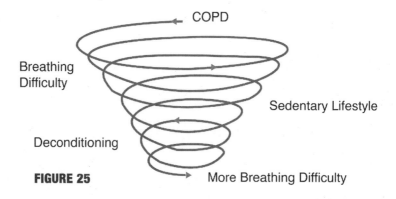

COPD

Breathing
Difficulty

Sedentary Lifestyle

Deconditioning

FIGURE 25

More Breathing Difficulty

The downward spiral of breathing difficulty leads to inactivity and deconditioning, which, in turn, can cause greater breathing difficulty.

To reverse this downward spiral, it is important that you begin some type of physical exercise. Although it is possible to do this on your own, participation in a pulmonary rehabilitation program offers many benefits.

Definition of Pulmonary Rehabilitation

"Pulmonary rehabilitation is a comprehensive intervention based on a thorough patient assessment followed by patient-tailored therapies that include, but are not limited to, exercise training, education, and behavior change, designed to improve the physical and psychological condition of people with chronic respiratory disease and to promote the long-term adherence to health-enhancing behaviors."[14]

A pulmonary rehabilitation program includes education and supervised exercise as well as support and encouragement. However, the most important part of a pulmonary rehabilitation program is exercise training, which directly improves your fitness and the efficiency of your muscles. Most hospitals or clinics in the United States have a pulmonary rehabilitation program this is paid for by health insurance and Medicare for individuals with moderate to advanced COPD. Typical activities are described below.

Typical Activities in a Pulmonary Rehabilitation Program		
	Arms	Legs
Aerobic	arm crank	walking on a treadmill
		pedaling on a stationary cycle
	elliptical machine	elliptical machine
Resisitance	stretch bands	resistance machine
	hand held weights	

In general, aerobic exercise will improve your overall fitness and endurance, while resistance training will improve your muscle strength. A rehabilitation specialist, usually a nurse or respiratory therapist, will monitor your heart rate and oxygen saturation while you do these activities. In addition, the rehabilitation specialist will:

- ask you to rate your breathing discomfort on a scale during exercise
- provide guidance and a reminder that it is okay to have some shortness of breath when you exercise
- evaluate whether you should use oxygen when you exercise
- instruct you on how to use pursed-lips breathing
- encourage you to pace yourself with activities

Another important feature of pulmonary rehabilitation is education. Topics usually include how to use inhalers, appropriate nutrition, coping skills, panic control, stress management, travel issues, breathing attacks, and sexual activity. Many individuals find psychosocial support, even just the ability to talk with others, quite helpful.

Benefits of Pulmonary Rehabilitation[15]

- improved exercise capacity
- reduced breathlessness
- improved quality of life
- reduced number of hospitalizations
- reduced anxiety associated with COPD
- improved strength and endurance of your arm and leg muscles

It may take a few weeks before you notice any of these benefits. Being able to breathe easier while doing certain activities should continue as long as you are motivated and work hard. Think about it as though you are an injured athlete training to regain fitness and stamina.

Most pulmonary rehabilitation programs ask that you attend two to three sessions per week for six to eight weeks. Hopefully, these six to eight weeks will be the start of a new lifestyle. Generally, you should plan to continue an exercise program to maintain the benefits. If you stop these activities after you complete the program, you will gradually lose the benefits of your hard work. Many pulmonary rehabilitation programs offer a maintenance phase in which you are able to use available exercise equipment but receive less monitoring and supervision.

Studies show that the effect of pulmonary rehabilitation on reducing breathing difficulty is generally much greater than achieved with use of inhaled bronchodilators. Along with using your maintenance COPD medications as prescribed by your doctor, you may wish to use an albuterol inhaler ten to fifteen minutes before starting each rehabilitation session.

You should discuss this with your doctor and the rehabilitation specialist.

Key Points

1. Over time, most people with COPD reduce physical activities to avoid feeling short of breath. This leads to deconditioning, or being out of shape.
2. Of all available treatments for COPD, pulmonary rehabilitation offers the greatest impact on improving your breathing and overall health.
3. Pulmonary rehabilitation programs include exercise training, education, and psychosocial support to help you make lifestyle changes.
4. After starting a pulmonary rehabilitation program, expect a few weeks to pass before you notice any improvements.

Follow-Up Vignette

The doctor referred Alice to the pulmonary rehabilitation program at the local hospital. When Alice started the program, she was somewhat anxious, but wanted to do everything the rehabilitation specialist suggested. For the first two weeks, she was tired after each session, and this fatigue carried over to the next day. Gradually, Alice noted that it was easier to do the various exercises and daily activities.

At the start of her fourth week in the program, the rehabilitation specialist told Alice that she was making excellent progress and recommended that Alice increase the incline on the treadmill by 1 percent and the resistance on the stationary cycle by 5 watts. Alice realized that the higher workloads would make the exercise somewhat harder, but that this change was necessary to improve.

CHAPTER 8

What Is a COPD Exacerbation?

Vignette

Bill is a fifty-nine-year-old man who was diagnosed with
COPD five years ago. He has been taking one long-
acting bronchodilator and has been able to do all of the activities of interest to him. Over the weekend, his daughter and
two young grandchildren came to visit. Both grandchildren
had chest colds and were coughing. A few days later, Bill
had a sore throat and his nose was congested. The next
day he started to cough and found that it was a little harder
to breathe when walking his dog. He began to use albuterol
twice a day for relief.

Over the next few days, he began to cough up yellow mucus,
and heard wheezing in his chest. One evening, he awoke at 2
a.m. with labored breathing. Bill felt like he was going to die,
and asked his wife to drive him to the Emergency Department
at the local hospital. When he arrived, Bill was found to have
a low oxygen level, and the doctor recommended that Bill be
admitted to the hospital for a "COPD exacerbation."

Introduction

The word "exacerbation" means a worsening or aggravation
of a problem. A COPD exacerbation means a flare-up or
sudden increase in one or more of the following symptoms:

- cough frequency or severity
- amount of mucus or change in color
- breathing difficulty

The following definition of a COPD exacerbation is used widely.

Definition of COPD Exacerbation

"A sustained worsening of the patient's condition, from the stable state and beyond normal day-to-day variations that is acute in onset and necessitates a change in regular medication."[16]

What Causes a COPD Exacerbation?

Most exacerbations (70–80 percent) are due to a respiratory infection that may be bacterial or viral. If the infection involves the airways, it is called acute bronchitis. If the infection involves the air sacs of the lung, it is called pneumonia.

A cause of 20–30 percent of COPD exacerbations is inhaling pollutants in the air. This may occur when the weather is humid and there is little air movement outside. These conditions are more common in the summer months in the northeast and Midwest of the United States. Some people describe the air as being heavy when the humidity is high.

Occasionally, it may be difficult for your doctor to determine the exact reason for your COPD exacerbation. Both heart failure and a blood clot in the lungs, known as a pulmonary embolism, may cause breathing symptoms that mimic an exacerbation.

Risk Factors for COPD Exacerbation

- older age
- daily cough productive of mucus (chronic bronchitis)
- another medical condition such as heart disease or diabetes

- heartburn (gastroesophageal reflux disease)
- a previous COPD exacerbation

In one study of over 2,000 patients, the single best predictor of having a COPD exacerbation was a history of a previous exacerbation.[17] Although you may not be able to change any of these risk factors, early recognition and treatment of an exacerbation should enable you to get better quicker. In general, your risk of having another exacerbation depends on the number that you had in the past year:

- **Low risk:** 0–1 exacerbation in the past year
- **High risk:** 2 or more exacerbations in the past year

How Do I Know If I Need an Antibiotic?

An antibiotic is generally prescribed if your doctor believes that it is likely you have a bacterial infection. How is this determined? Coughing up yellow or green mucus suggests a bacterial infection. The choice of a particular antibiotic depends on the severity of your COPD and any previous use of antibiotics in the past year or so. You may wish to discuss this with your doctor.

If you experience frequent chest infections or exacerbations, your doctor may prescribe an antibiotic for you to have available at home at the first sign of coughing up yellow or green mucus.

Will I Be Prescribed a Steroid for an Exacerbation?

When a COPD exacerbation occurs, the body increases the number of inflammatory cells in the airways in an attempt to heal. However, inflammation also causes the airways to narrow, which makes it harder for you to breathe (see Chapter 2). A steroid, which is short for corticosteroid, is frequently prescribed because it reduces inflammation and improves airflow.

If you are being treated at home, your doctor will likely prescribe a steroid pill called prednisone. The usual starting dose is 30–60 mg per day. Prednisone may be given for as few as five days or as many as fourteen days. Also, your doctor may tell you to reduce the dose every few days.

What Happens If I Am Admitted to the Hospital?

You may be admitted to the hospital if your breathing difficulty is bad enough or if your oxygen saturation is low. Usual treatments in the hospital include:

- bronchodilator medications inhaled from a nebulizer every two to four hours
- a corticosteroid given through a plastic tube placed intravenously; studies show that corticosteroids are effective in improving your symptoms and in decreasing the number of days you will spend in the hospital[18]
- an antibiotic if you have or are suspected to have a bacterial infection (acute bronchitis or pneumonia)
- a mask may be placed over your nose or over both your nose and mouth that is connected to a breathing machine if your breathing is quite difficult; the machine applies pressure to deliver air into your lungs, making it easier for your breathing muscles to work. This mask-machine system is called BiPAP, or bilevel positive airway pressure.

How Long Will the Exacerbation Last?

It is difficult to predict how long your symptoms of an exacerbation may last. Some individuals may feel back to normal in a few weeks. Others may continue to experience breathing problems and not feel well for one to two months. Most importantly, you should start to feel better after a few days of treatment and then hopefully continue to slowly improve. If you are not feeling at least somewhat better after two to three days of treatment, you should tell your doctor. Your doctor may ask you to come in for an appointment, or decide to wait and give the treatment another one to two days.

What Can I Do to Prevent an Exacerbation?

Fortunately, there are many actions you can take to reduce the risk of a future exacerbation. Certainly, you should stop smoking cigarettes if you were smoking before the exacerbation, and avoid inhaling irritants in the air. This includes staying away from secondhand smoke from family members and friends. You should be vaccinated for the flu virus every year and for pneumonia; the vaccine targets the most common bacterial cause of pneumonia called Streptococcus pneumoniae. Completion of a pulmonary rehabilitation program also reduces the risk of a COPD exacerbation.

In addition, three long-acting inhaled medications are approved by the FDA to reduce COPD exacerbations. These include tiotropium (brand name: Spiriva), fluticasone and salmeterol combination (brand name: Advair), and fluticasone furoate and vilanterol combination (brand name: Breo). See Chapter 4 for more information about these medications. Roflumilast (brand name: Daliresp) is a pill that also reduces the risk of an exacerbation, but only in those who cough up mucus on most days (a sign of chronic bronchitis) and have severe COPD. You should ask your doctor about these medications if you have frequent exacerbations.

Factors that Reduce the Risk of Another COPD Exacerbation

- quitting smoking
- avoiding irritants in the air, especially secondhand cigarette smoke
- vaccinations for the flu virus and pneumonia
- daily exercise on your own or pulmonary rehabilitation
- inhaled medications approved to reduce the risk: tiotropium, fluticasone and salmeterol, and fluticasone furoate and vilanterol
- roflumilast 500 mcg tablets once daily for those who have the chronic bronchitis type of COPD, severe airflow obstruction on breathing tests, and a history of exacerbations

In addition, long-term use of the antibiotic azithromycin taken three times a week can reduce the exacerbation rate in those who have experienced frequent exacerbations.[19]

What Is an Action Plan?

Many individuals who have COPD know when an exacerbation is starting because their symptoms tend to be similar to a previous exacerbation. If you have experienced one or more exacerbations, you should ask your doctor about an action plan. An action plan encourages you to begin treatment once you recognize that an exacerbation is starting. An action plan typically includes increased use of inhaled albuterol every four hours as needed, starting an antibiotic if you cough up yellow or green mucus, and possible early use of prednisone. Most doctors ask that you call their office once you've started the action plan to make sure that you are responding appropriately.

Key Points

1. A COPD exacerbation means a sudden worsening of symptoms, such as more frequent coughing, coughing up more mucus, coughing up yellow or green mucus, and more breathing difficulty.
2. Most exacerbations are due to a bacterial or viral respiratory infection.
3. The best predictor of having a COPD exacerbation is a history of previous exacerbations.
4. An antibiotic may be prescribed, especially if you are coughing up yellow or green mucus.
5. You can reduce the risk of having another exacerbation by stopping smoking, receiving flu and pneumonia vaccinations, participating in pulmonary rehabilitation, and taking one or more of the medications listed above.
6. You should talk to your doctor about an action plan if you have experienced one or more exacerbations in the past.

Follow-Up Vignette

Bill gradually improved after he was treated with an antibiotic, intravenous corticosteroids, oxygen, and nebulized bronchodilator medications. He was discharged after spending four nights in the hospital. He was relieved to be feeling better, and told his wife that "he was scared to death" the night that he awoke with breathing difficulty and went to the ED. His discharge instructions were to finish the antibiotic and taper the dose of prednisone.

At the appointment one week after discharge, the doctor reminded Bill that he must stay away from his cousin who was still smoking cigarettes, and reviewed appropriate hand hygiene with Bill and his wife. The doctor had his nurse give Bill the "pneumonia shot," as he had refused this vaccine previously. In addition, the doctor recommended that Bill start a long-acting beta-agonist combined with an inhaled corticosteroid inhaler to not only improve his breathing but reduce the risk of another exacerbation. Finally, the doctor referred Bill to the pulmonary rehabilitation program at the local hospital.

Although Bill felt a bit overwhelmed, he was happy that things were being done to improve his condition. The doctor said that he would schedule a follow-up appointment with Bill in one month and that they would discuss an action plan at that time.

CHAPTER 9

Will My Breathing Get Worse?
Will I Die from COPD?

Vignette

Betty is an eighty-two-year-old woman who has lived with COPD for fifteen years. She lives in an apartment with her cat, and is proud of her independence. She enjoys reading, spending time with her daughter and grandchildren, visiting with neighbors, and playing cards with friends. However, Betty is aware that it is getting harder to breathe when she does various activities, especially shopping, going to the hairdresser, and even spending time with her daughter's family. She knows that she tires easily.

Her COPD medications include a long-acting bronchodilator solution and a corticosteroid solution inhaled from a nebulizer twice a day, and two puffs of albuterol MDI used as needed. Six months ago, the doctor informed Betty that she needed to use oxygen at 2 liters/minute with activities and during sleep, but that she does not need oxygen when at rest.

After her brother-in-law died of colon cancer a few weeks ago, Betty started thinking about how her life might end. She decided to ask her doctor at her next appointment two questions: "Will my breathing get worse? Will I die from COPD?"

Introduction

Most of us don't like to think about getting older and dying. However, it is quite normal to think about our future, especially as we observe what happens to our family, friends, co-workers, and neighbors over the years. Some people want to know what is ahead, while others prefer to ignore this topic completely. It is important to remember what Lord Francis Bacon wrote over 400 years ago: "It is as natural to die as to be born."

Considering the end of your life in advance allows you to have some control of what will be done and what won't be done. It also provides an opportunity to consider what is important to you—your priorities.

This chapter describes what may happen to someone with COPD over time. However, it is important to remember three simple facts:

- No one has a crystal ball to predict the future.
- Your doctor can provide general information about COPD based on results of studies and his or her experiences.
- Each person is an individual and is on a unique journey.

Will My Breathing Get Worse?

This is a common question posed by individuals with COPD and their family members. Studies show that those with COPD generally report that their breathing difficulty slowly worsens over time. However, such reports reflect average changes and do not necessarily apply to each person with COPD. If your breathing difficulty is getting worse, it is very important to figure out why this is happening.

Why is this important? Because there is a good chance that whatever is causing your breathing to get worse can be treated, and if so, your breathing problem may improve.

Many patients with COPD assume, and often fear, that an increase in breathlessness is due to "my COPD getting worse." It is very important that you see your doctor in order to determine why your breathing is more difficult.

What should be done? First, breathing tests (PFTs) are needed to find out if your lung function has changed. If your test results are stable, you should consider the following possibilities: Have you gained weight? Are you out of shape? Do you have anemia (a low number of red blood cells)? Do you have heart disease? Are you anxious? Are you depressed?

Your doctor and possibly a pulmonary specialist can evaluate why your breathing is worse, and then recommend appropriate treatment.

Are There Treatments If My Breathing Gets Worse?

First, your doctor will make sure that you are using the best available bronchodilator medications (see Chapters 4 and 5) and will prescribe oxygen if necessary (see Chapter 6). If you continue to struggle to breathe at rest and/or with light activities, your doctor may ask if you would consider a trial of morphine.[20] Morphine is a narcotic medication used to treat pain and relieve breathlessness. Morphine works by changing the way the brain experiences breathing difficulty.

If you agree to try morphine, your doctor will most likely start you on a low dose that lasts for a few hours. If this provides some relief, your doctor may tell you to take one morphine tablet every four to six hours as needed. If the dose of morphine does not help you, your doctor will likely suggest a higher dose. Your doctor will help you adjust the dose and tell you how often to take morphine so that the breathing difficulty can be relieved. Your doctor will also tell you about possible side effects of morphine. The main concerns are sleepiness and constipation. Sometimes an anxiety medication is also recommended by your doctor because many individuals experience feelings of worry, tension, and fear when their breathing is difficult.

Will I Die from COPD?

The results of different studies provide general answers to this question.[21]

- If you have mild or moderate COPD, the main causes of death are lung cancer and cardiovascular disease (heart disease and stroke).
- If you have severe or very severe COPD, the main cause of death is that the lungs stop working. This is called respiratory failure.

Remember that this information applies to groups of people with COPD, and provides only a general idea of what may occur. Certainly, there are other possible causes of death for any of us, including pneumonia, blood clots to the lung, and cancers that start in other parts of the body, such as in the colon, breast, and pancreas.

What Is a Do-Not-Resuscitate Order?

A "do not resuscitate" (DNR) order means that cardiopulmonary resuscitation, or CPR, will not be performed if your heart or breathing stops. CPR involves someone pressing on your chest to help the heart pump blood, and someone breathing for you using either a bag system or mouth-to mouth. If a defibrillator device is available, or when an emergency medical technician (EMT) arrives, your heart may be shocked in an attempt to restart it. If you are not breathing on your own, the EMT will place a tube through your mouth into your windpipe, or trachea, to help you breathe. These actions are performed in an effort to keep you alive.

You may or may not have thought about whether you want CPR performed if an emergency occurs, and may wish to discuss with your doctor whether CPR would be beneficial for you or whether you would prefer a DNR order. Many individuals prefer not to think about these topics, which can be upsetting. However, if you are admitted to a hospital, your doctors are legally required to ask whether you want CPR. The reason for this is that if something happens to you suddenly as a hospital patient, CPR will automatically be performed. If you do not want CPR, the doctor will ask if you want to have a DNR order, which means that CPR and electric shocking of the heart will not be performed.

If you decide to have a DNR order, you will continue to receive all other treatments aimed at improving your health, including medications like oxygen and morphine to relieve your breathing difficulty.

You should also ask your doctor for a copy of the DNR order to have at home in case of an emergency. Make sure that family members are aware of your wishes and know where the copy of the DNR order is kept.

What Are Advance Directives?

All of us, whether healthy or ill, should have advance directives in case we become sick and unable to make medical care decisions. More than one out of four older Americans face questions about medical care near the end of life but are not able to make decisions because of an illness, an injury, or an inability to think clearly. An advance directive is a legal document that assigns the ability to make medical decisions for you to a trusted family member or close friend in the event that you are unable to do so.

To help guide this person, you should think about what kind of treatments you want or do not want if a medical emergency occurs. You should ask your doctor about what decisions you and your family might face if your COPD worsens. Talk to your spouse, children, and other close family members about your personal values and whether you favor staying alive as long as possible or value quality of life.

Tell your chosen decision maker about any activities (for example, being able to garden and spend time with family) and conditions (for example, living in your home rather than in a healthcare facility) that are important to you. That way, this person can share your wishes and goals with your doctors and the treatment team.

Advance directives include a living will and durable power of attorney for healthcare.

Advance Directives

Living will: A legal statement that informs your doctors about treatments if you are dying or unconscious and unable to make medical decisions. In a living will, you can describe which treatments you would want and those you do not want.

Durable power of attorney for healthcare: A legal statement that names a family member or friend to make decisions for you if you are unable to do so. This person should be familiar with your values and wishes about medical care, including a DNR order and whether you might be willing to donate any parts of your body.

If you decide you want advance directives, the next step is to fill out the legal forms that document your wishes. This may be done by a lawyer or a social worker, and many healthcare facilities have trained professionals available to assist you with the paperwork. In some states, your advance directive needs to be witnessed, and possibly your signature notarized. A notary is a person licensed by the state to witness signatures. A copy of your advance directives can be scanned into your electronic medical record in your doctor's office and at the local hospital.

You should tell your family members that you have completed advance directives, and give a copy to your healthcare proxy as well as your doctor. If you go to the Emergency Department or hospital for care, take a copy of these documents with you to be included in your medical records.

Key Points

1. Most of us don't like to think about getting older and dying. However, "It is as natural to die as to be born."
2. If your breathing is getting worse, you should tell your doctor so that he or she can determine whether your COPD is getting worse or whether there is another reason, such as weight gain, being out of shape, anemia, heart disease, anxiety, or depression.
3. Cardiopulmonary resuscitation (CPR) will be performed if you stop breathing or if your heart stops unless you have a "do not resuscitate" (DNR) order signed by a doctor.
4. You may wish to talk to your doctor about the details of a DNR order.
5. Consider advance directives, which include a living will and durable power of attorney for healthcare. Advance directives enable you to ask a trusted family member or friend to make medical decisions for you if you are unable to do so.

If you decide not to have advance directives and you become unable to make medical decisions, the legal system will determine who has authority to make medical decisions for you. In some states, your spouse, parents, and adult children, in that order, are your healthcare proxy by law. In other states, families must be in complete agreement with one another regarding any medical decision; otherwise a family member can petition the court system for the legal right to have authority for making medical decisions. Unfortunately, this process can create stress and tension in families if there is major disagreement about what should or should not be done.

It is important to remember that advance directives are only used if you are incapable of speaking for yourself and are in danger of dying and need treatment to keep you alive. A living will and durable power of attorney for healthcare allow you to continue to make your wishes known. Although completing advance directives can cause anxiety, hopefully the process will provide peace of mind for you and your family.

Follow-Up Vignette

At her appointment, Betty asked her doctor whether her COPD would get worse. Her doctor reassured her that some people with COPD can remain stable for a long time, and that it was impossible to predict the future course. The doctor reminded Betty that she should stay "as active as possible" and "continue to live with COPD."

The doctor asked Betty whether she had thought about CPR if she stopped breathing. At first Betty was upset by this question, but then realized it was necessary to think about this possibility. Betty knew that she did not want to be kept alive by a breathing machine. The doctor gave Betty some reading material that described the details of a "do not resuscitate" order. Betty said that she would read over the information and discuss it with her daughter.

The nurse suggested that Betty ask her daughter to come to her next appointment. The nurse also explained that advance directives were important for everyone whether you have COPD or not. The nurse informed Betty that advance directives would allow Betty to name someone like her daughter to make medical decisions for Betty if she was unable to make such decisions because of an illness or injury.

Later that day, Betty had a long phone conversation with her daughter. Betty's daughter agreed to go to the next appointment with her mother. At the appointment, the doctor discussed CPR and what a DNR order means. Betty said that she was ready for the doctor to sign a DNR order for her because she did not want CPR, a breathing machine, or her heart shocked. Her daughter said that she supported her mother's decision. Betty felt relieved after this was done.

Finally, Betty said that she needed to think about advance directives, and planned to discuss these with her daughter at a later time.

REFERENCES

1. Vestbo J, Hurd SS, Agusti AG, et al. Global Strategy for the Diagnosis, Management, and Prevention of Chronic Obstructive Pulmonary Disease: GOLD Executive Summary. *Am J Respir Crit Care Med*. 2013;187(4):347-365.

2. American Thoracic Society and European Respiratory Society. American Thoracic Society/European Respiratory Society statement: standards for the diagnosis and management of individuals with alpha-1 antitrypsin deficiency. *Am J Respir Crit Care Med*. 2003;168(7):818-900.

3. Parshall MB, Schwartzstein RM, Adams L, et al. An official American Thoracic Society statement: update on the mechanisms, assessment, and management of dyspnea. *Am J Respir Crit Care Med*. 2012;185(4):435-452.

4. Mahler DA, Harver A, Lentine T, Scott JA, Beck K and Schwartzstein RM. Descriptors of breathlessness in cardiorespiratory diseases. *Am J Respir Crit Care Med*. 1996;154(5):1357-1363.

5. Rennard S, Decramer M, Calverley PM, et al. Impact of COPD in North America and Europe in 2000: subjects' perspective of Confronting COPD International Survey. *Eur Respir J*. 2002;20(4):799-805.

6. Bauldoff GS, Hoffman LA, Zullo TG and Sciurba FC. Exercise maintenance following pulmonary rehabilitation: effect of distractive stimuli. *Chest*. 2002;122(3):948-954.

7. Mahler DA, Murray JA, Waterman LA, et al. Endogenous opioids modify dyspnoea during treadmill exercise in patients with COPD. *Eur Respir J*. 2009;33(4):771-777.

8. Gifford AH, Mahler DA, Waterman LA, et al. Neuromodulatory effect of endogenous opioids on the intensity and

unpleasantness of breathlessness during resistive load breathing in COPD. *COPD*. 2011;8(3):160-166.

9. Calverley PM, Anderson JA, Celli B, et al. Salmeterol and fluticasone propionate and survival in chronic obstructive pulmonary disease. *N Engl J Med*. 2007;356(8):775-789.

10. Tashkin DP, Celli B, Senn S, et al. A 4-year trial of tiotropium in chronic obstructive pulmonary disease. *N Engl J Med*. 2008;359(15):1543-1554.

11. Mahler DA, Waterman LA and Gifford AH. Prevalence and COPD phenotype for a suboptimal peak inspiratory flow rate against the simulated resistance of the Diskus® dry-powder inhaler. *J Aerosol Med Pulm Drug Deliv*. 2013;26(3):174-179.

12. Teip BL and Carter R. *Long-term supplemental oxygen therapy*. www.uptodate.com. 2014.

13. Stoller JK, Panos RJ, Krachman S, Doherty DE, Make B and Long-term Oxygen Treatment Trial Research Group. Oxygen therapy for patients with COPD: current evidence and the long-term oxygen treatment trial. *Chest*. 2010;138(1):179-187.

14. Spruit MA, Singh SJ, Garvey C, et al. An official American Thoracic Society/European Respiratory Society statement: key concepts and advances in pulmonary rehabilitation. *Am J Respir Crit Care Med*. 2013;188(8):13-64.

15. Casaburi R and ZuWallack R. Pulmonary rehabilitation for management of chronic obstructive pulmonary disease. *N Engl J Med*. 2009;360(13):1329-1335.

16. Rodriguez-Roisin R. Toward a consensus definition for COPD exacerbations. *Chest*. 2000;117(5 Suppl 2):398S-401S.

17. Hurst JR, Vestbo J, Anzueto A, et al. Susceptibility to exacerbation in chronic obstructive pulmonary disease. *N Engl J Med*. 2010;363(12):1128-1138.

18. Niewoehner DE, Erbland ML, Deupree RH, et al. Effect of systemic glucocorticoids on exacerbations of chronic obstructive pulmonary disease. Department of Veterans Affairs Cooperative Study Group. *N Engl J Med*. 1999;340(25):1941-1947.

19. Uzun S, Djamin RS, Kluytmans JA, et al. Azithromycin maintenance treatment in patients with frequent exacerbations of chronic obstructive pulmonary disease (COLUMBUS): a randomised, double-blind, placebo-controlled trial. *Lancet Respir Med*. 2014;2(5):361-368.

20. Mahler DA, Selecky PA, Harrod CG, et al. American College of Chest Physicians consensus statement on the management of dyspnea in patients with advanced lung or heart disease. *Chest*. 2010;137(3):674-691.

21. Sin DD, Anthonisen NR, Soriano JB and Agusti AG. Mortality in COPD: Role of comorbidities. *Eur Respir J*. 2006;28(6):1245-1257.

ABOUT THE AUTHOR

Donald A. Mahler, MD, is Emeritus Professor of Medicine at Geisel School of Medicine at Dartmouth in Hanover, New Hampshire. His current position is Director of Respiratory Services and pulmonary physician at Valley Regional Hospital in Claremont, New Hampshire.

While at Yale University School of Medicine, he developed the baseline and transition dyspnea indexes (BDI/TDI) in collaboration with the late Alvin Feinstein, MD, and colleagues. While at Geisel School of Medicine at Dartmouth, Dr. Mahler and the late John C. Baird, PhD, modified the BDI/TDI into self-administered computerized versions. These questionnaires are used widely in clinical trials of patients with COPD to assess the impact of new medications on breathing difficulty (dyspnea) with daily activities. The BDI/TDI have been translated into over 80 languages.

Dr. Mahler has written/edited four books on Dyspnea. The first was published in 1990, and the most recent was published in 2014 (CRC Press) co-edited with Denis E. O'Donnell, MD, of Queen's University in Kingston, Ontario, Canada.

He lives with his wife, Arlene, in Hanover, New Hampshire, and has four children and two grandchildren. He enjoys cycling, swimming, and growing basil to make pesto.